Towards MRCPCH
Part II (Theory)
Examination

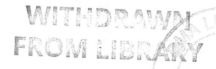

Towards MRCPCH
Part II (Theory)
Examination

Written by
Tapabrata Chatterjee
MD, MRCP (UK), MRCPCH (UK)
Paediatrician
Laurel Close, Grimsby
United Kingdom

Edited by
Suraj Gupte
MD, FIAP
Director, SOS Children's Health Centre
Professor and Head, Paediatrics II
Government Medical College, Jammu
Jammu and Kashmir, India

Hodder Arnold
A MEMBER OF THE HODDER HEADLINE GROUP

First published in India in 2004 by Jaypee Brothers, Medical Publishers (P) Ltd, EMCA House, 23/23B Ansari Road, Daryaganj, New Delhi 110 002, India

First published in the United Kingdom in 2005 by Hodder Arnold, an imprint of Hodder Education and a member of the Hodder Headline Group, 338 Euston Road, London NW1 3BH

http://www.hoddereducation.co.uk

This UK edition distributed in the United States of America by Oxford University Press Inc., 198 Madison Avenue, New York, NY10016 Oxford is a registered trademark of Oxford University Press

British Library Cataloguing in Publication Data
A catalogue record for this book is available from the British Library

Library of Congress Cataloging-in-Publication Data
A catalog record for this book is available from the Library of Congress

ISBN-10 [normal]   0 340 90584 0
ISBN-13   978 0 340 90584 5

1 2 3 4 5 6 7 8 9 10

Cover Designer: Nichola Smith

Typeset at   JPBMP typesetting unit
Printed at   Gopsons Papers Ltd., A-14, Sector 60, Noida

What do you think about this book? Or any other Hodder Arnold title? Please send your comments to www.hoddereducation.co.uk

Preface

All experienced clinicians in paediatrics, like other branches of medicine, have a system of pattern recognition in their mind, which often clinches the diagnosis or helps to approach a clinical problem.

Understanding this ever-recurring pattern is the basic philosophy behind advanced problem based learning. MRCPCH Part –II theory, tests this understanding of the common clinical scenarios of everyday life of a paediatrician.

I am including 50 gray cases and 75 data interpretation based on information of the candidates from their memory and my personal experience of the examination.

These questions are reconstruction of the themes from the basic philosophy of the questions that has come repeatedly in the examinations over a period of last five years. This book should also be a useful book for problem based learning for those who do not intend to take the MRCPCH examination. I have kept my discussions short, as this book is not intended to replace the comprehensive knowledge of common paediatric textbook, but an aid to apply the knowledge.

Tapabrata Chatterjee

Acknowledgements

I am grateful to my father Prof. Debabrata Chatterjee MD, FIAP who has helped me with his insight from his experience in paediatrics, particularly in neonatology and my mother Mrs. Dipti Chatterjee for her continuous support and motivation

I am extremely thankful to my wife Mrs. Barnali Chatterjee, for her enormous contribution in organising my work including all computer expertise and typing the whole manuscript, apart from her continuous inspiration and encouragement.

I would also like to thank my junior colleagues for letting me teach them and giving me the information from their examination experience, from which I could reconstruct the scenarios.

Finally I would like to thank Professor Suraj Gupte MD, FIAP for editing my book.

Contents

Data Interpretation
Questions 3
Answers 30

Gray Cases
Questions 51
Answers 84

How to Prepare for MRCPCH (Part II) Examination

MRCPCH Part II Examination consists of
- Theory
- Practical

The theory consists of
- Pictures ⎤ THEY ARE MIXED TOGETHER IN
- Gray Cases ⎬ TWO PAPERS
- Data interpretation ⎦ TWO AND HALF HOURS EACH

The practical consists of
- Long case
- Short case
- Viva

Pass marks
- At least 50% of total marks

HAVE TO GET AT LEAST 50% IN THEORY TO QUALIFY FOR PRACTICAL

- Have to pass in short case alone and long case and viva together (Long case can be compensated if there is bare fail only)

THEORY

Introduction

Qualifying marks to proceed to the practical 50%.

Generally 1ST impression is correct. Think twice before changing, even if tempted.

Use pencil

Make handwriting legible

Use capital letters like "TURNER'S SYNDROME"

Pictures

Generally half are photographic pictures and half are radiological pictures.

Tips

Read the questions and the written information provided with pictures. Most of the time, clue is there in the written information.

Look at the picture in a graded way:
  i. Look at the middle of the picture
  ii. Look at the side of the picture
  iii. Look at the surroundings (do not miss the father and mother if they are present with a child in a picture, as there might be useful clues to the diagnosis)
  iv. For a particular type of picture, think about the common possibilities

  Example – If a chest X-ray is given, think of
  Collapse of the lung
  Respiratory distress syndrome
  Bronchopulmonary dysplasia
  Cardiomegaly
  Rib fracture- non-accidental injury
  Diaphragmatic hernia
  Leaked TPN
  Pneumothorax

  v. Make a list before going for your examination like "CHEST X-RAY OF A ONE DAY OLD NEWBORN" causes include Group B sepsis, RDS, DIAPHRAGMATIC HERNIA, Meconium aspiration syndrome.

List will change if it is a 2 week old baby, a 4 week old baby or a two month old infant

vi. Do not forget to mention the side and try not to miss obvious adjectives; e.g.
Right- sided Erb's palsy instead of Erb's palsy
Right-sided tension pneumothorax instead of pneumothorax

Gray Cases

PREPARE AT LEAST 50 TYPICAL GRAY CASES. IF POSSIBLE 100 TO 150 CASES. PATTERN RECOGNITION IS MOST IMPORTANT.

Tips

i. Read the questions first before you read the text
ii. After that read the first sentence only and underline the age and the problem
iii. Read the investigation
iv. Form an opinion about the possible diagnosis
v. Read the whole text now

Example:
A 3-year-old Caucasian child who had prolonged jaundice in newborn period presents with abdominal pain. On examination he is pale and spleen tip is just palpable.
Investigation Hb-6 g/dl, Chest X-ray–normal.
Read the questions first before you read the text.
Q. What is the extra-abdominal cause of this abdominal pain?
Q. What further investigations are necessary to reach a diagnosis?
Q. What is the diagnosis?
You know that you are investigating a non-abdominal basic pathology causing abdominal pain.

Possibilities are
Pneumonia or referred pain from chest
Haemolytic process causing gallstone.

Go to the next part now. The first line may be
'This 3-year-old Caucasian child who had prolonged jaundice in neonatal period, now presents with abdominal pain.'
You already know that you are dealing with a haemolytic process in the Caucasian population.

Investigations:
Hb – 6 g/dl
Chest X-ray – normal
This child has got anaemia and the cause is not the chest. Thus without reading the text you can summarise your conclusion:
3-year-old
Anaemic child
History of jaundice
Haemolysis
Abdominal pain with non-abdominal pathology
Not chest related problem
Provisional diagnosis – **Hereditary spherocytosis** (do not write spherocytosis only)
Investigation – **Abdominal ultrasound** to rule out gallstone (do not write ultrasound).

Data Interpretation
AGAIN PATTERN RECOGNITION IS MOST IMPORTANT

Tips
  i. Read the questions first before you read the text.
  ii. After that read the first sentence only and underline the age and problem.

iii. Read the investigation.
iv. Form an opinion about the possible diagnosis.
v. Read the whole text now.

Commonly asked topics

ECG
Supraventricular tachycardia
WPW syndrome
ASD (Secondum type)
Prolonged QTc

EEG
Rolandic epilepsy
Absence seizure
Burst suppression of SSPE or Herpes encephalitis
Hypsarrhythmia

CARDIAC CATHETERISATION

FAMILY TREE - Like that of cystic fibrosis

AUDIOMETRY
Airborne gap- conductive deafness
Sensorineural deafness
Tympanometry

ACUTE RENAL FAILURE
Urinary parameters
Fractional excretion of Na
RENAL TUBULAR ACIDOSIS

MILK COMPOSITIONS

KARYOTYPING- Turner's, Down's, Trisomy 13,18.

BLOOD GAS – Do not forget to write the full result like – "partly compensated metabolic acidosis".

CSF – Picture of tuberculosis or partially treated pyogenic meningitis

50 to 60% of data is expected to come from this.

Tips

Lapse of concentration is cause failure in the theory examination. So be careful. Don't read anything the day before as that helps to preserve attention span. Best policy is to read the text and the questions at least twice and check your answers after writing as you get plenty of time.

Eventually, you are stuck at any part, leave that part and go to the next

Data
Interpretation

1.   ECG of a 6-year-old who was found to have bruit on routine examination.

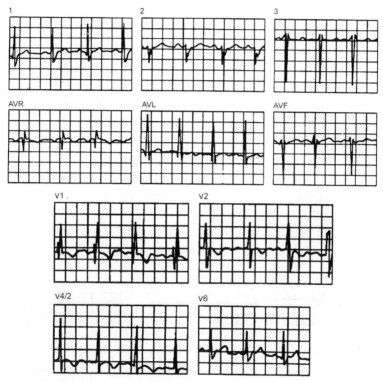

What is the likely cause?

2.   A 7-year-old with systolic bruit in second left intercostal space along sternal edge. Following results on cardiac catheterisation:

Partial pressure O$_2$:

SVC 64
IVC 68
RA 84 ↑
RV 83 ↟
PA 83 ↑

4 Data Interpretation

LA 96
LV 96

Manometric Pressures (in mm Hg):
RA 3
RV 55/2 ↑
PA 21/8 ↓
LA 4 ↓
LV 95/3 ↑

a) What abnormality is shown by the results?
b) What is heart lesion?

3. A child with headache, nuchal rigidity and low BP. CSF: lymphocytes ++, sugar low, chloride raised.
    Give 3 possible diagnoses.

4. ECG of an 8-year-old girl with goitre.

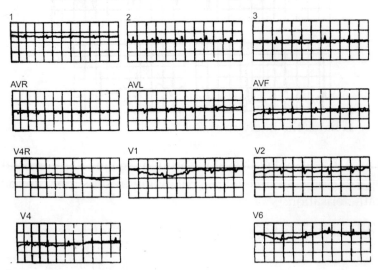

What is the diagnosis?

5. A 17-year-old male with pyrexia, vomiting, and photophobia of 3 days duration was treated with aspirin only. CSF: pressure 200, cells 30 (70% polymorphs, 30% lymphocytes), protein-100, sugar 60, no organisms on Gram stain.
  a) What is the most likely diagnosis?
  b) What are the 3 other diagnoses to be excluded?

6. A 9-day-old bottle- fed infant with convulsions.
  Plasma Ca – 1.2 mmol/l
  PO_4 – 1.0 mmol/l
  Alk phos – 1200 IU/L.
  a) How do the results explain the convulsions?
  b) Why might they have arisen?
  c) What is the significance of alkaline phosphatase?

7. A 3-year-old boy with heart failure and clubbing.
  pH – 7.46
  PCO_2 – 4.3 kPa
  PO_2 – 4.6 kPa
  HCO_3 – 28.

  a) What would be the expected FVC, FEV/FVC, CO transfer factor?
  b) Can O_2 be given safely?

8. A 6-year-old male presents with lumps in the groin and tiredness for 6 months.
  Hb – 11.8 g/dl
  MCHC – 32
  PCV – 37
  Retic – 2
  TWC – 150000
  L – 96%

6 Data Interpretation

N – 3%

E – 0.5%

a) What is the diagnosis?

b) Two serious complications other than infection?

9. A diabetic woman delivered a male at 36 weeks by caesarean weighing 3.4 kg. He became dyspnoeic 4 hours after delivery. Blood gas from umbilical artery catheter shows:

pH – 7.2

PO_2 – 5.2 kPa

PCo_2 – 8.5 kPa

HCO_3 – 30.

a) What is the diagnosis?

b) What two steps in treatment would you take?

10. A child can drink from a cup held by himself with two hands, say 2-3 word phrases, go by stairs one foot/ step with one hand held, build a tower of 3 using 2.5 cm cubes.

What is the developmental age?

11. A 2-day-old baby with birth weight 3.7 kg, at term had the following PO_2 value:

in air   4.55 kPa (35 mm of mercury)

100% O_2 6.55 kPa (50 mm of mercury)

Name two cardiovascular abnormality that commonly gives rise to this form of blood gases.

12. ECG of a 12- year-old boy who was found to have systolic murmur over pulmonary area.

a) What is the diagnosis?

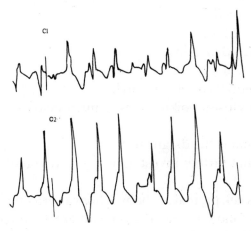

b) What symptom in such a patient is most important that you should ask?

13. A 6-year-old child had stridor for 2 hours.
    Chest X-ray – No thymus visualised
    Hb – 10.9g/dl
    WBC – 13.2
    N – 85
    L – 10
    B – 3
    E – 2
    Na – 136
    K – 4.3
    Cl – 107
    Ca – 1.9
    PO_4 – 2.2
    Urea – 4.
    a) What is the diagnosis?
    b) What further investigation would you perform?

14. A 3-year-old Pakistani boy had cough and wheeze.
    Hb – 11.7g/dl
    RBC – 5.2×10^{12}
    PCV – 0.355

MCV – 68 fl
MCH – 22.3 g
MCHC – 32.7 g/dl
WBC – 7.6 × 10^9/L
Differential count – normal,
Anisocytosis, poikilocytosis, microcytosis, and hypochromia.
a) What is the diagnosis?
b) What further investigation would you like to do?

15. A 33-week premature baby who was breathing on 100% O_2 had the following blood gas result at 8 hours of age:
pH – 7.07
PO_2 – 3.64 kPa (28 mm of mercury)
PCO_2 – 8.19 kPa (63 mm of mercury)
BE – 9.
What abnormality is present?

16. A 5-year-old presented with puffiness of the face and legs and smoky urine.
BP – 80/60
Urine dipstick – red cells ++, protein +++
Urine culture – negative
Serum albumin – 18 G/L
C_3 – Low.
What is the diagnosis?

17. A 26-year-old primigravida with diabetes mellitus, delivered a boy at 39 weeks of gestation weighing 3.5 kg. Child cried after birth and was pink. Baby was noted to be cyanosed and had respiratory distress at 18 hours of life. Arterial Blood Gas on oxygen with FIO_2 30%;
pH – 7.30
PCO_2 – 5.26 kPa (42 mm of mercury)
PO_2 – 6.5 kPa (50 mm of mercury).

What are the 2 diagnoses to explain the respiratory distress?

18. A 5-year-old Caucasian boy is noted to be pale and lethargic. He had a headache and stuffy nose for the past few days. He is known to have a big spleen for a long time. FBC shows:

Hb – 5.5 g/dl   TW – 6.7 × 10^9 differential count normal   Platelets – 100,000   Reticulocyte – 0.2%
Blood film – No blasts
PCV – 28
MCHC – 35
MCV – 86
ESR – 5
a) What is the diagnosis?
b) How can you explain the blood picture?

19. Father aged 46 years has myocardial infarction. Mother is worried and requests to screen the son for possible problem.

Serum cholesterol slightly raised -6.7 (normal-3 to 6.5)
What 2 laboratory investigations would you do?

20. Seventeen-months-old child with convulsion. Investigation including fasting test shows:

	Glucose	Insulin
0 hour	4.0	3.3
9 hours	3.5	3.2
18 hours	1.6	0

What is the diagnosis?

21. A 6-year-old girl with thirst; otherwise normal.
Investigations:
Urea – 3
Na^+ – 135
K^+ – 4

Ca^{2+} – 2.6
Blood sugar – 5.4
Urine microscopy and culture – normal
Early morning urine osmolality – 894 mosm/L
Early morning blood osmolality – 294 mosm/L.
How can you account for the increasing thirst?

22. A 6-year-old boy with severe headache, fever, vomiting for 5 days. No treatment was given. Neck stiffness noted.
    CSF: total cells 368 differential count L-98%, P-2%; protein – 1.5 g/L; sugar – 1.2
    Na^+ – 125
    K^+ – 3.0
    Urea – 2.0.
    a) What is the diagnosis?
    b) How can you explain the electrolyte values?

23. Two families with deafness:

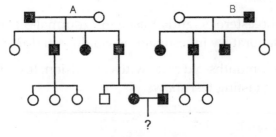

    a) What is this inheritance of A and B?
    b) What is the chance of a normal child if III (1) and (2) get married?

24. A 10-year-old boy had cough and fever for 3 weeks. He then developed neck stiffness and vomiting. CSF-cells 700-90% lymphocytes
    Pressure – 170 mm HG

Proteins – 1 g/l
Glucose – 1.5 g
Blood Glucose – 4.5 g
What two other investigations would you do on this CSF sample?

25. An 18-year-old girl with primary amenorrhoea and short stature. She is much shorter than her two sisters.
Hb – 10 g/dl
MCV – 110
Blood film-normochromic anaemia
Serum calcium – 2 mmol (corrected)
Serum phosphate – 0.9 mmol
Alkaline phosphatase – 900
a) What is the underlying diagnosis?
b) How do you explain the calcium and alkaline phosphatase values?
c) How do you explain the haematological abnormalities?

26. A 4-year-old acyanotic child with signs of cardiovascular disease. ECG given:

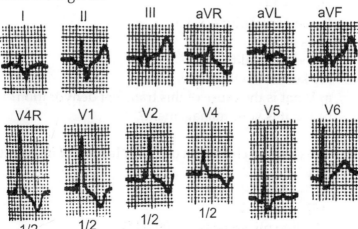

12   Data Interpretation

   a) List two abnormalities?
   b) What is the diagnosis?

27. Audiogram of child with Down's syndrome.

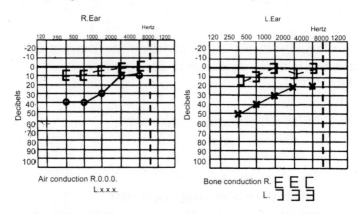

Air conduction R.0.0.0.
          L.x.x.x.

Bone conduction R. ⊑ ⊑ ⊏
              L. ⅃ ⅃ ⅃

   What is the diagnosis?

28. Baby 21 days old presented with signs of dehydration. Birth weight 1.7 kg, now lost 350 gm.

   Na – 165
   K – 4.5
   HCO_3 – 14
   Blood osmolality – 374.5
   Urea – 12
   Urine osmolality – 900
   No ketones in the urine.
   a) What is the cause of this transient dehydration?
   b) What is your management?

29. A 4-year-old child with one-year history of intermittent jaundice?

   ALT – 34 IU/L
   AST – 72 IU/L
   Alkaline phosphatase – 500 IU/L

Urine –   Urobilinogen negative
            Bilirubin positive.
a) What is the diagnosis?
b) What investigation would you do?

30. A 7-year-old girl has an abscess in a compound fracture.
    Grew *E.coli*
    Hb – 6.8 g/dl
    PCV – 28
    TW – 12.9 × 10^4
    Reticulocyte count – 5.5%
    Platelets – 75,000
    MCV – 87
    MCHC – 30.2
    Blood film – fragmented RBC
    Urea – 26, creatinine – 192
    Urine – RBC +++, protein + + +

    a) What is the haematological diagnosis?
    b) What findings did you base your results on?

31. Infant formula for 3 months. Is it appropriate?
    Calories – 67 cal/100 ml
    Protein – 1.3 gm%
    Fat – 3.7 gm%
    Carbonate – 7 gm%
    Sodium – 15 mg%
    Calcium – 33 mg%
    Phosphate – 15 mg%.

32. A 15-month old Sudanese child with fits.
    Calcium – 1.9 mmol/l
    Alkaline phosphatase – 1,500 IU/L
    Urea – normal.

14 Data Interpretation

   a) What is the diagnosis?
   b) What investigations would you suggest?

33. Lung function test on a 10-year-old boy with a one-month history of dyspnoea, FVC- decreased, FEV1/FVC - 85%. Total airway resistance increased.
   a) What is the abnormality?
   b) What is the diagnosis?

34. A 4-year-old Pakistani boy.
   Full blood count: microcytic hypochromic anaemia
   Hb – 5.9 gm/dl
   WBC, platelets – normal
   MCV – 85.
   a) What are the possible diagnoses?
   b) Give two confirmatory investigations.

35. A 6-week-old premature baby with birth weight of 1.5 kg.
   Hb – 8
   Reticulocyte count – 4%
   Peripheral smear – spherocytes and fragmented red blood cells.
   What is the diagnosis?

36. A 4-year-old asymptomatic girl was admitted for tonsillectomy. Routine urine test showed 1% glucose and trace of ketones. Her mother is a diabetic.
   Fasting blood sugar – 4.5 mmol/l
   Urine – 0.5% glucose
   What is the diagnosis?

37. A 5-year-old boy with cough.
   Full blood count – TW 27,000
   Lymphocyte – 70%
   What is the diagnosis?

38. A 2-year-old boy with generalised oedema.
    Urine protein – negative
    Serum albumin – low
    TW – 6,000
    Lymphocytes – 10%
    a) What is the diagnosis?
    b) Name two diagnostic investigations?

39. A 5-year-old child has haematuria and purpura
    Hb – 6.5 g/dl
    WBC – 6000, Neut – 1400, lymphocyte – 2800
    Platelet count – 15,000
    Blood urea and electrolytes – normal
    Choose the two most likely responses to explain the
    above changes?
    Acute lymphoblastic leukaemia
    Acute myeloblastic leukaemia
    Aplastic anaemia
    Induced aplasia
    Infectious mononucleosis
    Haemolytic uraemic syndrome

40. A 6-month-old girl presents with a two- month history
    of failure to gain weight.
    Sodium – 128
    Potassium – 3.2
    Urea –'7
    Bicarbonate – 11.
    Which single investigation is urgently needed?

41. Chromosomal analysis revealed the following karyotype
    in a 13-year-old girl.
    a) What is the diagnosis?
    b) How will be the intelligence of this child?

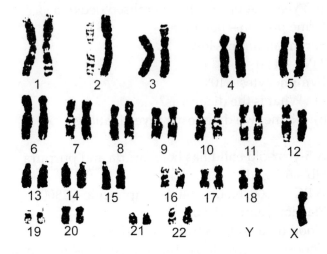

c) Give two drugs that the child should receive?

42.   This is an audiogram of a 6-year-old girl who was unable to speak even single words with meaning.

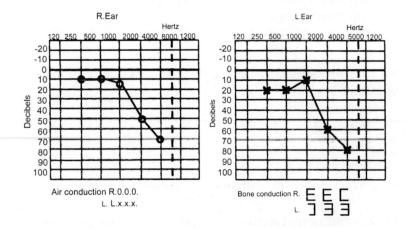

What is the cause of her inability to speak?

43. A 7-year-old girl presented with nose bleed. The following laboratory results were obtained:

Full blood count – Normal
Platelet count – Normal
Prothrombin time – Normal
APTT – 60 s (control 42 s)
Thrombin time- normal
Factor VIII C – 20%
Factor VIII R – Ag – 25%
Bleeding time – 15 min (control 5 min)
Platelet aggregation to ristocetin – reduced
What is the mode of inheritance?

44.

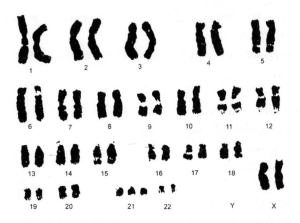

This is the karyotype of a newborn baby with dysmorphic feature. This child is vomiting since birth and therefore on IV fluids. He has also been noted to have a heart murmur.

a) What is the likely cause of vomiting?
b) What will the abdominal X-ray show?
c) What is the commonest cardiac lesion causing murmur in this child?

45. A 3-year-old Caucasian child presents with fever and bloody diarrhoea. After 3 days the diarrhoea resolves but child became aneuric.
Investigation shows:
Hb – 9 g/dl
White cell count – 12 × 10⁹/l
Platelet count – 40 × 10⁹/l
Plasma potassium – 7.6 mmol/l
Plasma sodium–128 mmol/l
Plasma urea – 16.3 mmol/l
Blood film – Polychromasia, schistocytes and toxic granulation
Activated partial prothrombin time – 40 s (38 s in control)
Prothrombin ratio 1.1
a) Why is this child aneuric?
b) What further blood test that you can do to confirm the cause of anaemia?
c) How would you bring down the high potassium immediately?

46. A two and half-year-old with waddling gait. Started to walk at 13 months. On normal diet.
Investigations:
Ca^{2+} – Normal
PO_4^{2+} – 0.6
Alkaline phosphatase – 320
Parathyroid hormone – 0.6 ng (normal < 0.9 ng)
Dehydrocholesterol – 20 (normal)
Urea normal – 3.8
Creatinine – 30
a) What is the diagnosis?
b) Name two therapeutic agents.

47. A 12-year-old boy with recent onset of epistaxis.
    Hb – 7.2 g/dl
    PCV – 0.3
    Reticulocyte – 6.2%
    Platelet count – 190,000
    BT – 15
    CT – 5
    Factor VIII assay 20%
    a) What is the diagnosis?
    b) What drug to avoid?

48. Pedigree chart showing affected boy with achon-droplasia. He has a normal sister and parents are normal.

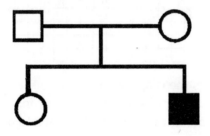

    a) What is the risk of parents having another achondroplastic child?
    b) If sister marries a normal male, what is the risk?

49. A 2-month-old child, Hb-5.5 g/dl, WBC- 10,000, platelet-400,000.
    a) What is the clinical diagnosis?
    b) How will you confirm?

50. This ECG was taken immediately after birth of a newborn baby whose mother was suffering from a systemic illness.

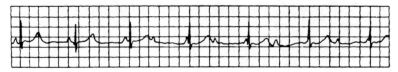

What is the illness of the mother?

51. A 3-year-old boy was referred by the GP because of shortness of breath. In the GP letter, GP mentioned that though the chest sounds clear, he was unable to count the pulse rate. ECG was taken at admission.

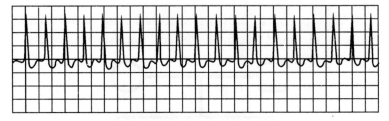

   a) What is the diagnosis?
   b) An intravenous medicine was instituted and the child's heart rate immediately went back to normal. What is the medicine?

52. The karyotype is reported as 45XX t (14,21). The parents want to know the result of the investigation. What will tell them?

53. A 6-year-old presented with fever for 10 days. Initially treated by GP with ampicilllin. Examination showed slight neck stiffness and mild hemiparesis.
   CSF data:
   Protein – 800 mg/dl
   Sugar – 0.7 mmol/1(RBS 4.2)
   WBC – Nil

Culture – No growth
Total count – Not high.
   What is the probable diagnosis?

54. This is a growth chart of a baby born at term. He was doing well till four and half months. During this period he was on exclusive breastfeeding. Solids were introduced at around this time but the child developed irritability, palor and diarrhoea. Some investigations were done at around 8 months of age and dietary modifications lead to improvement of child's status.

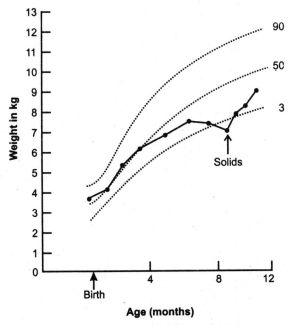

Age (months)

   a) What investigation made us suspect about the diagnosis?
   b) What investigation confirmed the diagnosis?
   c) What dietary modification cured the child?

55. Cardiac catheterisation for a 12-year-old boy:

% Saturation	Pressure (mmHg)
SVC	68
RA	68
RV	68
PA	68
LA	98
LV	8
Aorta	95

What is the cardiac diagnosis?

56. Bilateral audiogram:

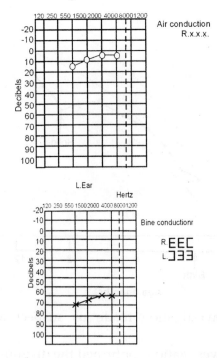

What is the diagnosis?

57. This is a family tree of a child who had delayed motor milestones and became wheelchair bound by the age of 10 years.

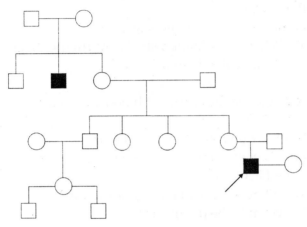

a) What is the mode of inheritance?
b) What is the diagnosis?

58. A 17-year-old boy referred for short stature. He also complains of tiredness. Father and a 14 -year-old brother have appropriate height. Father 5′ 9″, mother 5′4″, brother 5′6″.

Examination: pale, height 5′2″, weight 40 kg. Unbroken voice. No secondary sexual character. He has small genitalia, blood pressure is normal. No other physical abnormality.

Investigation:
    Hb – 8 g/dl
    MCV – 98
    MCHC – 27
    Urine microscopy and culture – normal
    ALP – slightly raised
    AST – normal
    ALT – normal

ESR – 3
Serum bilirubin – 12 mmol/L
Ca^{2+} – 2.25
PO_4 – 0.84
Urine – no albumin, no sugar.
a)   What investigation shall confirm the diagnosis?
b)   What is the diagnosis?

59.   A 2-year-old boy, arterial blood gas on air.
pH – 7.35
PCO_2 – 7.8 kPa (60 mm of mercury)
PO_2 – 7.8 kPa (60 mm of mercury)
Total HCO_3 36
a)   What is the acid base abnormality?
b)   What is the diagnosis?

60.   Child can copy

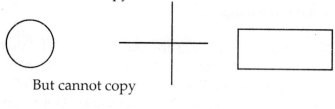

But cannot copy

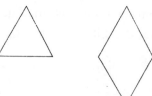

What is the age (single age)?

61.   A 16-year-old girl lives with flat mate, found by flat mate comatose. She had 5-day history of vomiting, nausea, abdominal pain right upper quadrant.

O/E RR 120, BP 88/40, jaundice, responsive to pain stimuli. Deranged APTT/PT/ INR---, BM 2.8, transaminase ---i, HCO_3; 24, EEG- generalized slow waves.

Tick the most appropriate answer:

a) What is the most likely diagnosis?
   A. Alcohol ingestion
   B. Paracetamol o/d
   C. Aspirin

b) What are the most significant prognostic factors?
   A. EEG
   B. Transaminase
   C. APTT
   D. Prothrombin time
   E. Glucose

62. A 3-month-old child in the community with concerns over weight gain. Mum fed three and half scoops of powdered milk mixed in 105 ml of boiled water.

What will be your advice?

63. A newborn male baby continued bleeding at site of fetal electrode on day 1 of life.

Hb – normal
Plt – normal
APTT – 100 (control 30)
PT – normal

What is the likely diagnosis?

64. A 1½-year-old child presents with diarrhoea and not putting on weight.

Na – 128
K – 3.5
Cl – 98
HCO_3 – 11
Urea – 24
Serum osmolality- 330

What other biochemical investigations you need urgently?

65. Boy walked at 13 months of age.
    Development normal
    $Ca^{2+} - 4$
    $PO_4 - 0.7$
    ALP – 1200
    LFT – normal
    pH – 7.35
    Urine pH – normal
    Urine amino acid – negative
    25-Vit D – normal
    What is the most likely diagnosis?

66. A boy who is 14-year-old, in puberty, known epileptic,
on carbamazepine for 2 years.
    FBC – normal
    ALP – 400 (150-200 adult level)
    Other liver transaminases normal.

    What is the likely reason for the increased ALP?

67. A 5-month-old child presents with jaundice, diarrhoea,
vomiting.
    U and E normal
    Bili – 1.8 mmol/l
    Urine – reducing sugar – 1.4 mg/l
    Urine – no glucose, no blood, no protein.

    What investigation would you do to help with diagnosis?

68. This is an EEG from a 6-month-old child who was being
investigated for abnormal movements of his head, legs and
arms.
    a) What is the diagnosis?
    b) What is the initial drug of choice?

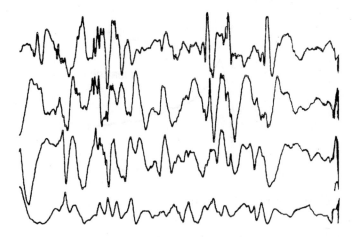

c) What is the drug of choice if the child is unresponsive to the initial treatment?

d) What is the problem with the second medication?

69.

A

B

C   V4R   V6

Can you determine the approximate age of three healthy children with the ECGs above?

70. This is the DTPA scan of a 5-month-old baby whose antenatal scan showed dilatation of renal pelvis.

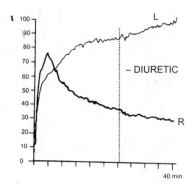

Comment on the scan.

71. This 10-year-old girl has vacant episodes.

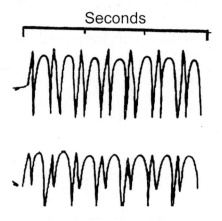

What is the diagnosis?

72.

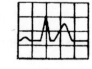

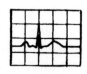

A and B are the ECGs of a child before and during the treatment of diabetic ketoacidosis. A intervention was done and after that ECG C was obtained after 12 hours of ECG B.

a) What are the abnormalities in ECG **A** and **B**?

b) Institution of what treatment led to ECG **C**?

73. The following results are obtained from a 2-year-old boy who has not passed urine for 12 hours. This urine sample was obtained after catheterisation of bladder. Urine osmolality – 600 mmol/L. Urinary sodium – 10 mmol/L.

a) What is the likely cause of aneuria in this child?

b) What will be the likely fractional excretion of Sodium?

74. A one-year-old child who was born with a birth weight of 3 kg at 38 week of gestation, was 7 kg at the end of one year. Investigations revealed:

HCO_3 – 10

Serum sodium – 138

Serum potassium – 5

Serum chloride – 120

Urinary pH – 5.5

Urine also showed generalised glycosuria, phosphaturia, and aminoaciduria.

a) What is the cause of acidosis in this child?

b) What is the most common cause?

75. A 14-year-old boy was investigated for an episode of renal colic. Urine microscopy showed:

RBC – high

WBC – high

Urine culture – no growth, hexagonal crystals present

Abdominal X-ray – radio opaque shadows

Urine cyanide nitroproside test – positive

a) What is the likely diagnosis?

b) What would urine amino acid chromatography show?

c) What treatment is required?

Answers

1. Atrial septal defect, ostium primum.
   Discussion: Right bundle branch block pattern presents with RSR pattern in the right-sided chest leads (V_1 and V_2). Right bundle branch block pattern with left axis deviation as shown in the ECG occurs in ostium primum, atrial septal defect or AV canal defects. Never comment about ventricular hypertrophy if there is bundle branch block pattern. If there was right bundle branch block pattern with right axis deviation, we should have been thinking of secondum type of atrial septal defect.

2. a) Raised right ventricular pressure; step up in oxygen saturation in right atrium.
   b) Pulmonary stenosis with atrial septal defect.
   Discussion: If there is a step up or step down in the oxygen saturation, at a particular level, the shunting is at that level. If there is decrease of pressure from one chamber or vessel to another, this denotes stenosis.

3. Tuberculous meningitis, Partially treated pyogenic meningitis, Viral meningitis.
   Discussion: Lymphocytic preponderance in the CSF can occur in tubercular meningitis, viral meningitis and partially treated or early stages of pyogenic meningitis.

4. Hypothyroidism
   Discussion: This type of ECG showing low voltage trace can also occur if there is incorrect standardisation, in obesity, in pericardial effusion, in constrictive pericarditis, and in hypopituitarism.

5. a) Bacterial meningitis.
    b) Cerebral abscess; early tuberculous meningitis; cryptococcal meningitis.
    Discussion: It is important to note that just as in early bacterial meningitis we can get lymphocytic response, in early tubercular and viral meningitis, we may get a neutrophilic response.

6. a) Hypocalcaemia
    b) High phosphate diet
    c) None.

7. a) All decreased.
    b) Yes.
    Discussion: Heart failure and clubbing can occur either in a chronic respiratory illness or in a congenital cyanotic heart disease. However in a congenital cyanotic heart disease there is acidosis and not alkalosis, due to decreased tissue oxygen delivery. Therefore this picture describes a chronic respiratory illness like cystic fibrosis where we may get hypochloraemic, hypokalaemic alkalosis (pseudobartter syndrome).

8. a) Acute lymphoblastic leukaemia.
    b) Intracranial bleed, thrombosis secondary to hyper-viscosity, hyperuricaemia.
    Discussion: In a 6-year old boy lymphadenopathy with very high total count is suggestive of acute leukaemia though non-Hodgkin lymphoma may also be considered. Intracranial bleed can occur in acute lymphoblastic leukaemia even with a comparatively higher platelet count compared to conditions like ITP where intracranial bleed is very rare even with a very low platelet count. Tumour lysis syndrome is a dreaded

complication of ALL especially after initiation of treatment. Priming with allopurinole and monitoring the electrolytes are necessary.

9. a) Respiratory distress syndrome.
    b) Surfactant administration
        CPAP or positive pressure ventilation
    Discussion: This is a big baby born to a diabetic mother, which denotes poor diabetic control. Infant born to a diabetic mother are prone to respiratory distress syndrome even when they are near-term or term. The blood gas picture shows evidence of respiratory acidosis with some degree of metabolic compensation so typical of a baby with respiratory distress syndrome.

10. 18 months to 2 years.

11. Transposition of great arteries (TGA)
    Pulmonary atresia

12. a) Wolff-Parkinson-White (WPW) syndrome
    b) Palpitations.
    Discussion: Pattern recognition is very important for interpretation of an ECG. In an apparently normal ECG, it is important to look for δ wave, wide QRS complex and short PR interval. WBW syndrome is the commonest cause of supraventricular tachycardia, which presents with palpitations as a symptom.

13. a) Hypocalcaemia due to hypoparathyroidism.
    b) PTH assay, chromosome for microdeletion.
    Discussion: Hypocalcaemia with elevated phosphorus but normal urea makes us think of the diagnosis of hypoparathyroidism. Absence of thymic shadow in the

chest X-ray at this age, may signify absence of thymus. The constellation of hypoparathyroidism and absence of thymus should alert us towards the diagnosis of DiGeorge syndrome.

14. a) Iron deficiency
    b) Serum ferritin assay.
    Discussion: Iron deficiency anaemia is the commonest cause of microcytic anaemia in any child. Serum ferritin estimation can confirm the diagnosis. Low ferritin can occur even before haemoglobin falls significantly.

15. Hypoxia with mixed respiratory and metabolic acidosis.
    Discussion: Low pH denotes acidosis. As CO_2 is high there is respiratory component. As base excess is < -5, there is metabolic component. This type of picture in a premature baby is typical of respiratory distress syndrome, where surfactant deficiency leads to inadequate CO_2 clearance and, therefore, respiratory acidosis. Inadequate lung expansion also causes hypoxia. Tissue hypoxia leads to metabolic acidosis.

16. Nephritic onset of nephrotic syndrome.
    Discussion: Low albumin with proteinuria confirms the diagnosis of nephrotic syndrome. The commonest cause of nephrotic syndrome in childhood is minimal change glomerulonephritis. However, presence of haematuria and low C_3 makes minimal lesion unlikely. The causes of a low C_3 in a child with glomerulonephritis are acute poststreptococcal glomerulonephritis, membranous glomerulonephritis and membrano proliferative glomerulonephritis.

17. Idiopathic respiratory distress syndrome.
    Group B- Streptococcal pneumonia.

Discussion: Respiratory distress syndrome, is not uncommon in infants of a diabetic mother even when they are term. Such a baby may be born pink and normal at birth but subsequently becomes tachypnoeic. Blood gas described above shows evidence of mild respiratory acidosis. As it is impossible to differentiate RDS from Group B pneumonia either clinically or radiologically, it is usual that these babies are covered with antibiotics till 48 hr culture results come back.

18. a) Hereditary spherocytosis.
    b) Aplastic crisis due to parvovirus infection.
    Discussion: Persistent isolated splenomegaly in a Caucasian child is hereditary spherocytosis unless proved otherwise. Anaemia with low reticulocyte count, low platelet and lowish total count denotes aplastic picture. Aplastic crisis is common in hereditary spherocytosis when there is a parvovirus B19 infection.

19. Lipoprotein electrophoresis, serum triglyceride level.

20. Ketotic hypoglycaemia.
    Discussion: Ketotic hypoglycaemia is the commonest cause of non-hyperinsulinaemic hypoglycaemia in a child.

21. Psychogenic
    Discussion: When there is polyuria and polydipsia and increasing thirst, we should think of five differential diagnosis.
    1) Diabetes mellitus
    2) Central diabetes insipidus
    3) Nephrogenic diabetes insipidus

4) Chronic renal failure
5) Psychogenic polydipsia
As the blood sugar is normal, this cannot be diabetes mellitus. As the urea is normal, this is not chronic renal failure. In Diabetes insipidus, body cannot concentrate urine adequately due to lack of (central) or insensitivity to (nephrogenic) antidiuretic hormone. However, in this child the early morning urine is concentrated in spite of normal blood osmolality. Therefore, this is not central or nephrogenic diabetes insipidus. Thus, the polydipsia in the 6-year old girl is of psychogenic origin.

22. a) Tuberculous meningitis.
    b) Dilutional effect due to syndrome of inappropriate ADH secretion.
    Discussion: Insidious onset of raised intracranial pressure, together with lymphocytic leukocytosis, high protein and low sugar in CSF in untreated child points towards a diagnosis of tuberculous meningitis. Tuberculosis is on an increase all over the world, after the epidemic of HIV. Lymphocytic leukocytosis in the CSF, suggests diagnosis of tuberculous meningitis in a child with febrile illness and neck stiffness and high protein and low sugar helps to differentiate it from viral meningitis. SIADH is common at presentation in any form of meningitis.

23. a) Autosomal dominant-Family A and B
    b) Like that of normal population.
    Discussion: As all generations are affected the deafness in family A and B are of dominant inheritance. As there is male to male transmission of deafness in both the families, the deafness is autosomal. There is many autosomal dominant deafness that exist in any

population. Therefore, it is unlikely that these two families will have same autosomal dominant deafness.

24. Acid fast bacilli in the CSF
    CSF adenosine deaminase activity
    CSF, PCR for *Mycobacterium tuberculosis*

25. a) Coeliac disease
    b) Malabsorption of vitamin D
    c) Folic acid deficiency
    Discussion: Primary amenorrhoea and short stature in a 18-year-old girl makes us suspicious of coeliac disease and Turner's syndrome. However, anaemia and hypocalcaemia with raised alkaline phosphatase point towards rickets, which is more likely to occur following malabsorption in coeliac disease.

26. a) Incomplete right bundle branch block pattern
        Right axis deviation.
    b) Ostium secondum atrial septal defect.
    Discussion: Right bundle branch block pattern presents with RSR pattern in the right-sided chest leads (V_1 and V_2). Right bundle branch block pattern with left axis deviation as shown in the ECG occurs in ostium primum, atrial septal defect or AV canal defects. Never comment about ventricular hypertrophy if there is bundle branch block pattern. If there was right bundle branch block pattern with right axis deviation, we should have been thinking of secondum type of atrial septal defect.

27. Bilateral conductive hearing loss due to glue ear.
    Discussion: Recurrent glue ear is extremely common in children with Down's syndrome. The presence of the airborne gap in audiogram signifies conductive deafness.

28. a) Neonatal transient diabetes mellitus.
    b) Correct dehydration, administer insulin.
    Discussion: Osmolality is calculated by the formula $2(Na+K)+$ urea+glucose. Hypernatraemia can occur due to injudicious fluid containing high sodium (generally oral) administration, diabetes mellitus and diabetes insipidus. In a 21-day-old neonate, injudicious oral fluid administration is unlikely. Diabetes insipidus is ruled out because the urine is concentrated. The calculated osmolality on the basis of the formula $2 (Na+K) +$ urea +glucose gives a glucose value of 23.5. Therefore, the diagnosis is transient neonatal diabetes mellitus. The syndrome of transient diabetes mellitus in the newborn infant has its onset in the first weeks of life, and persists only for several weeks to months before resolving spontaneously. It occurs most often in infants who are small for gestational age and is characterised by hyperglycaemia and pronounced diuresis with glycosuria resulting in severe dehydration and metabolic acidosis with minimal or no ketonuria.

29. a) Choledochal cyst.
    b) Ultrasound abdomen.
    Discussion: Choledochal cyst is the commonest cause of intermittent conjugated hyperbilirubinaemia.

30. a) Microangiopathic haemolytic anaemia due to haemolytic uraemic syndrome.
    b) *E.coli* infection, peripheral blood film, low Hb, high reticulocyte count, low platelet count, high blood urea and creatinine.
    Discussion: *E.coli* 0157 liberates toxins which causes haemolytic uraemic syndrome. This commonly follows

a bloody diarrhoea due to *E. coli*. However, *E. coli* infection elsewhere in the body can also precipitate renal failure. Pneumococcal infection can also produce haemolytic uraemic syndrome. However HUS following pneumococcal infection is rare.

31. Appropriate.

32. a) Rickets.
    b) X-ray hands.
    Discussion: Hypocalcaemic tetany can uncommonly occur in children with rickets.

33. a) Obstructive and restrictive lung function.
     b) Cystic fibrosis.
     Discussion: Cystic fibrosis leads to fibrosis and bronchiactatic changes resulting in the restrictive pattern. Wheezing and increased airway resistance is also universal in cystic fibrosis and therefore we get a mixed picture.

34. a) Iron deficiency anaemia.
     b) Serum ferritin, haemoglobin electrophoresis.
     Discussion: Microcytic hypochromic anaemia may occur due to iron deficiency or due to haemolytic anaemia like thalassaemia. Serum ferritin will be low in iron deficiency and high if there is haemolytic process. Haemoglobin electrophoresis will show abnormal haemoglobin bands in haemoglobinopathies.

35. Anaemia of prematurity.

36. Renal glycosuria
     Discussion: Stress-induced hyperglycaemia and glyco-suria due to diabetes mellitus would have caused

glycosuria with high blood sugar. However, in this child the blood sugar is normal. Therefore, renal glycosuria could be the only possible explanation for glucose in the urine.

37. Whooping cough.
    Discussion: Paroxysmal cough with absolute lympho-cytosis is a feature of whooping cough, though similar picture can occur rarely in some viral infections (like adenoviral infection). Pertussis immunisation does not always give full immunity though undoubtedly makes the disease milder.

38. a) Protein-losing enteropathy due to intestinal lymphangiectasia.
    b) Chromium level albumin studies, blood α_1 anti-trypsin level, jejunal biopsy.
    Discussion: In intestinal lymphangiectasia the absolute lymphocyte count is low and there is a nephrotic syndrome type of picture without proteinuria.

39. a) Acute lymphoblastic leukaemia
    b) Aplastic anaemia
    Discussion: Pancytopenic presentation of acute lymphoblastic leukaemia, though uncommon, is not unheard of. As the condition is so common compared to other conditions in the list, it deserves a high position in the differential diagnosis. Aplastic anaemia (being also quite common) should come in differential diagnosis. Haemolytic uraemic syndrome (HUS) can also present with anaemia and thrombocytopenia but because blood urea is normal the diagnosis of HUS can be ruled out.

40 Serum 17- hydroxy progesterone assay.
   Discussion: Salt-losing crisis with acidosis is a common feature of congenital adrenal hyperplasia.

41. a) Turner's syndrome
    b) Normal
    c) Growth hormone and oestrogen.
    Discussion: Turner's syndrome in children have normal intelligence as far as IQ is concerned. However, in a recent study it is shown that there is increased incidence of attention deficit hyperactive disorder (ADHD) in children with Turner's syndrome. Replacement therapy with oestrogen is indicated along with growth hormone therapy, but there is little consensus about the optimal age at which to initiate treatment with oestrogen.

42. Bilateral, partial sensorineural deafness.
    Discussion: The audiogram shows high frequency loss in air conduction, which is more characteristic of sensorineural than conductive deafness.

43. Autosomal dominant.
    Discussion: In von Willebrand's disease, both bleeding time as well as coagulation profile will be abnormal. Though factor VIIIC is abnormal, both in classical haemophilia and in von Willebrand disease, factor VIIIR:Ag will be normal in classical haemophilia. Therefore, diagnosis of von Willebrand disease,which has got autosomal dominant inheritance will be appropriate in this scenario.

44. a) Duodenal atresia
    b) Double bubble appearance.
    c) Atrio-ventricular septal defect.
    Discussion: This is the picture of a child with Down's syndrome with karyotype (47XX+21).

45. a) Acute renal failure due to haemolytic uraemic syndrome

b) Peripheral blood smear which will show fragmented RBC.

c) Nebulise salbutamol.

Discussion: *E. coli* 0157 infection causing bloody diarrhoea is the commonest cause of haemolytic uraemic syndrome in the UK. Nebulise salbutamol has been found to be an effective in acutely reducing hyperkalaemia.

46. a) Hypophosphataemic rickets.
    b) High dose vitamin D/analogues and phosphate supplements.

47. a) von Willebrand's disease.
    b) Aspirin

Discussion: Von Willebrand disease and not classical haemophilia is the appropriate answer in this scenario as both bleeding time and factor VIII is abnormal. In classical haemophilia though the factor VIII assay will be abnormal, bleeding time will be normal.

48. a) 1 in 50,000.
    b) Risk will be slightly more than that of normal population.

Discussion: Although neither parents are affected, the risk of having another affected child is above the general population as one of the parents may exhibit gonodial mosaicism.

49. a) Diamond-Blackfan syndrome
    b) RBC adenosine deaminase assay, bone marrow aspiration.

Discussion: Low haemoglobin in a child of this age with normal WBC and platelets is suggestive of pure red cell aplasia. The reticulocyte count also is low in this condition.

50. Maternal systemic lupus erythematosus (SLE).
    Discussion: Complete heart block in a newborn can be an isolated finding, can be associated with structural abnormalities of heart like transposition of great arteries, and can occur following cardiac surgery. However, as mother was suffering from a systemic illness, maternal SLE will be the most likely cause of this condition in the present scenario.

51. a) Supraventricular tachycardia
    b) IV adenosine.
    Discussion: IV adenosine, which needs to be given in form of rapid bolus IV injection, can dramatically restore the heart rate to normal in supraventricular tachycardia.

52. Balanced Robertsonian translocation for Down's syndrome. The child is phenotypically normal but a potential carrier of Down's syndrome
    Discussion: If the karyotype was 46 XX t (14,21), the child would have fitted into the diagnosis of Down's syndrome due to unbalanced Robertsonian translocation. Translocation occurs in 2-3% of the individuals with Down's. The most frequent translocation is Robertsonian 14,21 translocation as described in the karyotype given. In this form the carrier would have one 14 chromosome, one 21 chromosome, and one fused 14,21 chromosome giving a total of 45 chromosome and they are phenotypically normal. However, when a carrier produces offspring there is risk of producing unbalanced karyotype. The likelihood of female carrier producing an unbalanced trisomic child is 15% and the likelihood

of male carrier producing an unbalanced trisomic child is 2.5% in the karyotype shown in the picture.

53. Partially treated meningitis with subdural effusion; cerebral abscess.

54. a) Coeliac screen
    b) Jejunal biopsy
    c) Gluten-free diet.
    Discussion: In a child who started failing to thrive after introduction of solids makes us suspicious of clinically coeliac disease. Coeliac screen for antigliadin and antiendomysial antibiotics makes the suspicion stronger, jejunal biopsy confirms the diagnosis and gluten free diet helps in curing the child with catch up growth.
    A similar growth chart is often asked in the examination where a child fails to thrive at around 8-9 years and thyroxine treatment (after appropriate diagnostic investigation of hypothyroidism) cures the condition.

55. There is some difficulty to explain the stepping up of oxygen from LV to aorta. Apart from this, most of the candidates agreed with the diagnosis of tetralogy of Fallot, post palliative shunt.

56. Left-sided profound sensorineural deafness.
    Discussion: This deafness is profound both as it is present both at high frequency as well as in low frequency. This means the child is almost unable to hear anything on the left side.

57. a) X-linked recessive.
    b) Duchenne-muscular dystrophy

Discussion: This is a predominantly muscular problem as evidenced by delayed gross motor milestones. The family tree did not show any male to male transmission and spared generations. Therefore the mode of inheritance is X-linked recessive. The most common X-linked recessive muscular problem is Duchenne's muscular dystrophy

58. a) Triple anterior pituitary stimulation tests.
    b) Panhypopituitarism.

59. a) Compensated respiratory acidosis.
    b) Cystic fibrosis/Adenoidal hypertrophy.
    Discussion: Obstructed sleep apnoea can cause compensated respiratory acidosis and, therefore, difficult to distinguish from cystic fibrosis from blood gas picture. However, overnight SaO_2 monitoring and sweat test will confirm our diagnosis.

60. 4 ½ years.

61. a) Paracetamol overdose.
    b) Prothrombin time.
    Discussion: As paracetamol is available over the counter in the UK. Paracetamol overdose is the commonest overdose for deliberate self harm.

62. Increase the amount of feed to approximately 150 ml/kg of the expected weight.

63. Classical haemophilia.

64. Blood sugar.
    Discussion: Calculated osmolality 2(Na + K)+Urea + glucose. Blood sugar according to this formula, 43 as

serum osmolality is 330 and Na is 128, K is 3.5, urea is 24. Therefore, diabetic ketoacidosis is the likely pathology in this scenario as bicarbonate is also low.

65. X-linked dominant hypophosphataemic rickets.

66. Pubertal growth spurt.

67. Galliput test.

68. a) Infantile spasm
    b) ACTH
    c) Vigabatrine
    d) It can cause visual field defects, which is difficult to monitor at this age.

69. **ECG A** – Newborn
    ECG B – Infant (1 month to 1 year)
    ECG C – Older child and adult
    Discussion: If we see a newborn ECG pattern in a older child or adult we should think of right ventricular hypertrophy. Similarly if we see the adult ECG pattern in a newborn baby we should think of left ventricular hypertrophy.

70. Right sided pelvico-ureteric function is normal. However in the left side there is pelvic dilatation due to obstruction either in the pelvico-ureteric or vesico-ureteric function.

71. Absence seizure.
    Discussion: Classical 3 per second spike wave pattern confirms the diagnosis of absence seizure, which may sometimes be precipitated by hyperventilation.

72. a) ECG **A** – shows tall T waves suggestive of hyperkalaemia.
    ECG **B** – shows flat or dyphasic T waves suggestive of hypokalaemia.
    b) Addition of potassium to the IV fluid solved the problem and ECG **C** is a normal ECG.
    Discussion: Before treatment the serum potassium in diabetic ketoacidosis may be high, though the total body potassium is invariably low. Starting of treatment with insulin there is rapid internalisation of potassium inside the cells. This may result in severe hypokalaemia. Therefore, it is important to add potassium to IV fluids while treating DKA once the urine output is established.

73. a) Dehydration
    b) Les than 1%.
    Discussion: In patients with hypovolemia, the urine is concentrated and the fractional excretion of sodium is less than 1%, by contrast, in patients with tubular necrosis the urine is dilute (osmolality < 350) and the sodium concentration usually exceeds 40 and the fractional excretion of sodium exceeds 1%.

74. a) Proximal tubular acidosis due to Fanconi's syndrome
    b) Cystinosis
    Discussion: Anion gap= (Na+K) – (Cl+Bicarbonate). Normal anion gap in presence of metabolic acidosis can occur only in renal tubular acidosis. As the urinary pH was 5.5 it means that urine could be acidified to lower value than 6 unlike distal tubular acidosis, where urine pH is always above 6. The presence of aminoaciduria, glycosuria and phosphaturia denotes that the cause of this proximal renal tubular acidosis is Fanconi's syndrome. Cystinosis is a common cause of Fanconi's

syndrome and the severe failure to thrive in this child is likely to be due to the development of chronic renal failure related to cystinosis.

75. a) Cystinuria
    b) Cystine, ornithine, lycine and argenine (remember COLA)
    c) High fluid intake, sodium bicarbonate to form alkaline urine, D- penisalamine, surgical intervention for stones.

   Discussion: The hexagonal crystals and positive cyanide nitropruside test in the presence of radio-opaque calculi raises the suspicion of cystinuria. Urinary amino acid chromatography confirms that diagnosis.

Gray Cases

1. A 14-year-old girl presents with backache of 3 days duration. Over the past 24 hours she has developed progressive weakness of her lower limbs and complains that her face feels puffy. Subsequently she had noticed that her arms feel weak and she finds it difficult to lift them above her head.

In her past medical history she had meningitis at the age of 6, which resolved completely and since then has been well with only occasional upper respiratory tract infections. She is fully immunised including BCG.

On examination she is fully oriented but has flaccid weakness of both lower limbs and can barely raise them off the bed. The tendon reflexes are elicitable in the legs. Both planters are flexor. In addition she has weakness of both arms and bilateral weakness of the facial muscles.

Hb – 13 g/dl
WCC – 7
Plts – 300
U and Es – normal
LFTs – normal
LP – normal

a) What is the likely diagnosis?
b) What is the next most important investigation?

2. A 15-year-old girl presents with a 6-week history, initially starting with swelling and tenderness of the right ankle, and subsequently developed erythema nodosum. She also suffered with malaise, fever, night sweats and some abdominal pain.

Her past medical history is uneventful, and she is fully immunised including BCG.

When she was seen, she was noted to have lost weight and also developed pharyngeal ulcers.

Hb – 13 g/dl

WCC – normal
Red cell indices – normal
U and Es – normal
ESR – 49
Rheumatoid factor – negative
LFTs – normal
Mantoux – 1:1000 5mm erythema at 48 hours
24 hour protein excretion normal.
a)   What is the most likely diagnosis?
b)   What is the best confirmatory investigation?

3.   A 2-year-old boy presented with facial swelling and oedema, ascites, scrotal oedema, and proteinuria. Urinalysis shows albumin ++++. His blood pressure was 80/45, pulse 100/min and respiratory rate at 20/min. There was no blood or white cells in urine and the urine culture is negative. The remainder of the examination is normal.
Hb – 18 g/dl
WCC – 11
Plt's – 540
Na – 130
K – 5.8
Urea – 15
Creatinine – 280
Albumin – 12
ASO titre – negative
24 hour urine protein excretion – double the normal.
Over the next 3 days his urea rose to 21 and his creatinine to 320.
a)   What is the diagnosis?
b)   What is the likely cause for his deterioration in renal function?

4. A 27-year-old a Rh positive woman was in her second pregnancy with twins. The pregnancy had been uneventful and she had been healthy. At 29 weeks gestation she went into spontaneous labour. There was no prolonged rupture of the membrane. Of the twins, one was delivered vaginally, weighing 1.36 kg, with good Apgar scores and needed no initial resuscitation over the next four hours of life. The baby developed grunting and sternal recession, and required 18 hours of maximum 30% incubator oxygen.

The second of the twin presented with a cord prolapse, developed a poor cardiotocograph with prolonged decelerations, and was delivered by emergency caesarian section, 15 minutes later. She arrived in poor condition, pale and apneic, was intubated and given the dose of surfactant and needed prolonged ventilatory support and intensive care management.

a) What is the cause of respiratory problem in the first twin?

b) What is the cause of respiratory problem in the 2nd twin?

5. A 15- year-old boy with history of fever, headache and rash. He had been well until the day before when he developed a headache, and pain on moving his eyes. On the day of admission he developed fever and rash. He also developed swelling of fingers and a painful swollen ankle. There was no significant illness in the past. The family and the social history were normal. On examination he was fully conscious and oriented. Temperature was $38.4°$ C. Pulse 120/min. BP 90/50 mm of Hg. There was no neck stiffness and any focal neurological signs were absent. The hand was swollen with a vasculitic rash. The rash was seen on the arms, legs and over the eyelids. There was no splinter haemorrhages. The interphalangeal joints of the 4th and 5th digits of the right hand and the 3rd and 4th and 5th of the left hand and the right ankle joint were swollen and tender.

Hb – 12.1 g/dl

WBC – Polymorphonuclear leucocytosis

Platelet count – normal

Urine – No proteins or glucose

Blood urea and electrolytes – normal

a) What is the investigation that will allow you to make your diagnosis?

b) What is the diagnosis?

c) What two steps would you take immediately?

6. A 10-year-old girl was admitted with a history of pain in her legs and refused to bear weight for the last 3 days. The past history, family history and social history were all normal. She has been fully vaccinated. There has not been any travel abroad.

On admission she was apyrexial. There was weakness of both lower limbs, left side was more than the right. Proximal muscles were weaker than the distal muscles. Reflexes were absent on the left side, and reduced on the right side. Plantars were flexor. Sensations were normal. There was no tenderness over the back. All other systems were normal. Over the next few days in hospital she developed weakness of her upper limbs and urinary retention. On the 5th day after admission she complained of difficulty in breathing.

a) What is the likely diagnosis?

b) What immediate therapeutic step would you take now?

7. A baby weighing 2.6 kg was delivered by forceps at 39 weeks of gestation, due to deceleration on the CTG detected during the 2nd stage of labour. Baby developed some respiratory distress and was given bag and mask ventilation to which it responded very well. At 3 hours of age he developed prolonged apnoeic episode but was found pink immediately afterwards. He then became progressively tachypnoeic, developed expiratory grunt and intercostal and subcostal recessions. The other systems were normal on examination.

Hb – 17g/dl

WBC – 6,000

Platelet count – 95,000

Chest X-ray – ground glass appearance with air bronchogram.

What is the most likely diagnosis?

A. Group B Streptococcal (GBS) sepsis

B. Heart failure

C. Surfactant deficiency

D. Transient tachypnoea

E. Inborn error of metabolism.

8. A 15-year-old boy is brought to you because of small stature. His parents are fairly sure that growth was much the same as his peers until 8 years of age. His general health has been good, appetite normal and, apart from morning headaches over the past few months, there has been no symptoms and no significant past history of consequence. He attends the local secondary school where he is of average ability, but he is not keen on sports.

The father is 178 cm tall and was pubertal about the age of 13 years. The mother is 152.4 cm tall; her menarche was at 15 years. There is one 14-year-old male sibling, who is taller than his brother.

Examination:

Height – 140 cm (<3rd centile)

Weight – 34 kg (<3rd centile)

No secondary sexual characteristics, infantile penis, both testes of prepubertal size.

All other systems normal.
a)   What clinical examination would you do?
b)   What imaging study may be helpful?
c)   What is the diagnosis?

9.   A 5-year-old boy, 2-3 history of cough, which is loose cough, worse in morning and after exercise and 2 isolated episodes of wheeze. Few courses of antibiotics from a GP showed some improvement. Salbutamol MDI 200 μg QDS for 6 months showed no improvement.

Mum has epilepsy, 1 sibling has eczema. In the past there was recurrent otitis media from 7 months.

On examination:

Weight < 3rd centile, height 25th centile.

Looks well, no other abnormality on examination, except bilateral crackles in the chest.

Chest X-ray shows right lower lobe bronchial shadowing on 3 occasions over 6 months.

Sweat Test	Weight	120 mg
	Na	28
	Cl	23

Sputum Haemophilus on 2 separate occasions
IgG lower range of normal
IgA, IgM, IgE all normal
FBC and Diff normal
ESR-18.

a) What is the underlying respiratory disease?
b) What investigation would you do to confirm this?
c) What 2 investigations would you do to confirm the underlying diagnosis?

10. A 4-month-old baby girl presented with a 3- day history of poor feeding, vomiting, irritability. She was born by caesarian section at 36 weeks. BW 2.6kg, weight today – 5 kg. Mum is from Tanzania, Black African, Dad is a Caucasian civil engineer.

On examination:
Pale, tachypnoeic (66/min), subcostal recession, cervical lymphadenopathy, palpable lymph nodes, liver and spleen. There was marked oral candidiasis and she deteriorated and required intubation and ventilation.

Chest X-ray : Bilateral patchy opacities, air bronchiogram and hyperinflation.

FBC – normal, lymphocytosis, albumin 28, Total protein- 80

Virology (RSV, adenovirus, influenza, etc) negative
Commenced on IV cephalosporin.

a) What investigation would you do to confirm the respiratory diagnosis?
b) What investigation would you do to confirm the underlying diagnosis?
c) Which two of the following would you give?
   A. IV hydrocortisone
   B. IV gancyclovir
   C. IV cotrimoxazole
   D. IV metronidazole
   E. IV amphotericin
   F. IV gentamicin
   G. IV frusemide
   H. IV albumin

11. A girl presented at the age of 3 ½ years with excessive thirst and polyuria. The blood glucose was normal. A diagnosis of diabetes insipidus was made and she was treated with regular deamino arginine vasopressin (DDAVP) per nasally. Her control was always difficult and deteriorated as she got older, necessitating several hospital admissions. Her behaviour was a major problem, but her mother was devoted and accompanied her on each admission, administered the DDAVP and checked the urine specimens.

By the age of 8 years her weight was on the 3rd centile, height 40th centile and urine osmolality around 250 mmol/kg with a serum Na^+ level of 140 mmol/l, K^+ 4 mmol/l, urea 4 mmol/l, and Ca^{2+} 2.2 mmol/l. During an admission to try and improve her control, the mother had to attend a sudden bereavement in the family. This resulted in the child having a tantrum and refusing all medication. That evening the serum osmolality was found to be 295 mmol/kg and urine 420 mmol/kg.

a) What is the diagnosis?

b) How do you confirm this?

12. A 4-day-old, exclusively breast fed baby was noted to be pale, with heart rate of 180 with gallop rhythm, palpable liver of 2 cm and black sticky stools. Baby was born in an ambulance, from where she was transferred to post-natal ward. Pregnancy was uneventful, but delivery was quick. This was mother's fourth child. Baby was discharged home after 24 hours.

a) What 2 investigations would you do to establish your suspected diagnosis?

b) What 2 therapeutic interventions would you undertake?

c) What is the diagnosis?

13. A 15-year-old boy presented with a history of foul bulky diarrhoea, with onset while on holiday in Russia. A number of classmates also had similar symptoms. He had a past medical history of pertussis as a child and had been left with a productive cough producing yellow green sputum on most

days during winter. He had also been admitted to another hospital after a mass was found in the right iliac fossa at a routine school medical. A laparotomy had been performed and a normal appendix removed; in addition a dilated caecum which had been opened and the contents evacuated. On examination his weight was between the 10th and 25th centile and his height between the 25th and 50th centile. There were early signs of puberty. He had bilateral basal crackles on respiratory examination. On abdominal examination, there was a non-tender mass on right iliac fossa. Apart from clubbing, examination was otherwise normal.

Other investigations:
Full blood count – Normal
ESR   – Normal
Electrolytes   – Normal
Jejunal biopsy   – Normal
Chest X-ray   – Normal heart size. Bilateral shadowing
Faecal fat   – Marked raised

a) What diagnostic investigation would give the most information?
b) What is the underlying diagnosis?
c) What is the cause of the right iliac fossa mass?

14. A 3-year-old boy was brought in, who awoke screaming that morning with apparent right lower quadrant pain. He had been previously well with an entirely normal past medical history. He was pyrexial and flushed. On examination he had a temperature of 39.4°C. His right hip was internally rotated and slightly flexed with pain on passive movement. Passive movement of the knee and ankle on the right side and all joints on the left leg were normal with a full range of movements. Abdominal examination revealed 2 cm hepatomegaly. He was drinking normally but had watery diarrhoea.

Investigations:
Full blood count – Hb 10.9 g/dl, WCC – 28 × 10^9/1 (84% neutrophils)
Platelets – 390 × 10^9/1
ESR – 110 mm/hour
Abdominal X-ray – Normal
X-ray hips – Normal
   a) What 3 initial investigations would you arrange?
   b) What is the diagnosis?

15. A 5-year-old boy who started walking at 18 months of age presented with a 2-year history of difficulty in walking. His mother had noticed that he had been worse over the last month. In addition he had a rash over his face and hands, which had been diagnosed as eczema over the last 6 months but had not responded to steroid creams. There was a history of maternal uncle with myasthenia gravis. He gave a history of difficulty in walking up the stairs, inability to get up from the floor without holding onto furniture and some neck weakness. On examination he had neck weakness, ankle jerks were present, other reflexes were difficult to elicit.
a) What is the diagnosis?
b) Name one investigation, which is the most likely to confirm the diagnosis?

16. A 7-year-old boy of Turkish Cypriot origin was admitted. He was born and brought up in the UK. He had been on a 3 weeks holiday to Cyprus, having returned one week ago, during which time he enjoyed the local diet including shell fish. He presented with a 24- hour history of pallor, jaundice and brown- red urine and normal stool.
   Hb – 7.9 g/dl
   SBR – 50 µmol/l

a)   Give two diagnoses you could think of as differential guide to further questioning?
b)   What is the cause of the urine colour for each of the answers?

17. A girl aged 5 presented with a 3-week history of lethargy and bruising. She had also history of pains in the feet and legs. She had suddenly deteriorated over the previous 24 hours and started vomiting and was dehydrated.
Investigations:

> Hb – 7 g/dl
> White cell count – $3.0 \times 10^9/1$
> Platelet count – $5 \times 10^9/1$
> Urea – 40 mmol/l
> Creatinine – 140
> Uric acid – raised

a)   What are the two most likely causes of the renal failure?
b)   What are the 2 most important investigations?
c)   What is the most likely underlying diagnosis?

18. A 15-year-old girl who had VSD repaired at 18 months of age, when the pulmonary and aortic pressures were equal. She was well since but with reduced exercise tolerance, especially compared with twin sister who had a small VSD requiring no intervention.

Six weeks back, at annual check up she was in sinus rhythm, with a rate of 80.

Over the next 3 weeks she became breathless with ankle swelling and on the day of admission had an episode of chest pain and haemoptysis.

On examination –
Slightly cyanosed, tachycardic and breathless.
Ankle and sacral oedema

JVP raised at 7-8 cm
Chest – Crepitations bilaterally
Heart sounds – loud P2, diastolic murmur upper left sternal edge.

ECG showed atrial fibrillation

a)   What caused the haemoptysis on the day of admission?
b)   What precipitated the episode of being unwell for the preceding 3 weeks?
c)   What is the cause of her heart failure?
d)   What is the cause of chest pain?

19.   A 9-year-old Caucasian boy was admitted following a 7-day history of cough, high temperature and abdominal pain. On examination he was pale, icteric with injected tonsils and had a tender abdominal mass below the left costal margin.

Investigations:
Hb – 4.2 g/dl
MCV – 60 fl
Total white cell count – $1.1 \times 10^9/l$
Neutrophils – $0.6 \times 10^9/l$
Platelets – $85 \times 10^9/l$
Reticulocytes – 2%
Direct Coombs test-negative
Total bilirubin – 110 µmol/l
Unconjugated bilirubin – 95 µmol/l
Urinalysis – no abnormality detected

a)   What is the diagnosis?
b)   What investigations would help to confirm this?
c)   What probable complication has arisen?

20.   The newborn baby of a diabetic mother, taken to Special Baby Care Unit at 5 minutes of age – with mild cyanosis,

audible systolic murmur at lower level of left sternal edge, and metabolic acidosis. Baby was ventilated. Chest X-ray showed cardiomegaly, with a poor view of lungs.

Give 2 cardiac lesions causing this picture?

21. A 2-year-old boy has recently stopped walking and became pale and miserable. He complained of limb pains. On examination a mass left hypochondrium extending to midline, 4 cm liver, no splenomegaly.
a)   Give 3 investigations you would do?
b)   What is the most likely diagnosis?

22. A 5-year-old boy with a 2-week history of fever was generally unwell and lethargic with maculopapular rash on the face and trunk. Two days later he complained of hip pain and held the hip extended and externally rotated. Over the next few days, he developed intermittent fever, but no splenomegaly or lymphadenopathy.
Investigations:
    FBC – normal
    ESR – 7
    Hip joint aspiration – clear effusion, few white cells and red cells only.
    Hip X-ray – NAD
    Bone scan – NAD
    What is the likely diagnosis?

23. A 16-year-old girl, previously well, wakes suddenly during the night with fever, headache, shivering, diarrhoea and vomiting. No significant past history except innocent heart murmur as a child. She was not on any medication. On arrival to the hospital, he was noted to have petechiae across abdomen and sunburn-like rash in the groin area. Blood pressure was 80/45, he was icteric with deranged LFTs.

   a) What is the diagnosis?
   b) Give 3 possible aetiological factors?

24. A 16-year-old Italian girl with hereditary spherocytosis had splenectomy done 3 months ago. She was admitted with fever for the past three days. Two days prior to admission, she was noted to have a painful swelling over her left ankle, which later involved the right ankle and the right elbow.

Investigations:
   Hb – 10.6 g/dl
   WBC – 20,000/ml (neutro 80%)
   Platelets – 230,000/ml
   Peripheral blood film – spherocytes +++, Howell-Jolly bodies and normoblasts.
   a) What are the 2 investigations that you would like to do?
   b) What is the most likely diagnosis?
   c) Name two measures that would prevent this occurrence?

25. A 15-year-old girl was admitted via Accident and Emergency Department with periorbital swelling, lip and tongue swelling for 12 hours. She had developed abdominal pain with vomiting 6 hours ago and was noted to have stridor for past 2 hours. She had a similar episode one year ago after a bee sting. This had resolved after one day. There was no family history of allergies.

   On examination, the periorbital, tongue and lip swelling were noted. There was inspiratory stridor, but no crackles or rhonchi. BP- 120/80 and pulse rate- 100/min.
   a) What is the cause of the stridor?
   b) What is the underlying diagnosis?
   c) What two immediate treatment that you would do?

26. A 2-year-old boy was admitted with 3-day history of fever and generalised rash. He received two doses of

amoxycillin, after which rash appeared. He was treated by a
GP for fever and sore throat. The amoxycillin was stopped
after the rash appeared.

On examination:
Temperature -39° C
Conjunctivitis present
Red lips with some cracking
Pharynx injected with modest tonsillar nodes
enlargement. Erythema of hands.

Initial investigations:
Hb – 11.2 gm/dl
Raised total count
Platelets – 273,000/ml
Septic screen
After 6 days in the hospital, the fever persisted in spite
of IV antibiotics. The septic screen was negative. The chest
was clear and the Chest X-ray was normal. Investigations
were repeated.
Hb – 10.8 gm/dl
Raised – TW
Platelets – 730,000/ml
ESR – 138 mmHg
a) What is the one investigation that you would like to do?
b) What is the most likely diagnosis?

27. A 6-year-old boy sustained injury to his right shin after
being kicked during a game of football. Over the last 2 days,
he had fever, malaise and pain over the medial aspect of his
right thigh. He refused to weight bear or walk. He has a past
medical history of meningitis at the age of 3 years and has
learning difficulties in school. Otherwise, no other medical
complaints. His two siblings were well.

On examination:

   T – 38° C

   Right hip in flexed position

   Abrasion over the right shin

   Tenderness on the medial aspect of the right thigh and groin and the lower abdomen above the inguinal ligament. He resented movements of the right hip because of considerable pain.

   The left hip and the left side of the abdomen was normal.

Investigations:

   Urine protein and microscopy normal

   FBC showed raised total count

   Chest, Abdomen and X-ray of right hip/femur were normal.

a)   What two investigations would you do?

b)   Give two most likely diagnoses.

28. A 6-year-old girl referred after school medical examination noted her to be tall for her age. She was delivered by full term normal vaginal delivery at term with birth weight of 3.2 kg. No past medical illness of significance. No history of vaginal bleed either. Mother's height was 168 cm and father's height was 188 cm. A maternal aunt was tall for her age as a child.

Social history is of no relevance.

On examination:

   Height – 149 cm (below 97th centile)

   Weight – 36 kg (below 97th percentile)

   Breast development – palpable breast tissue

   Fine pubic hair but no axillary hair.

   The rest of the physical examination including the pulse rate was normal.

a)   What is the most likely diagnosis?

b)   What are the next 3 investigations that you would do?

29. A 30-week gestation baby with a birth weight of 3.2 kg developed cyanosis and respiratory distress at 15 min of life. He was ventilated and put on IV dextrose infusion and was pink and stable on ventilator.

Ventilator settings – pressure 20/3
Inspiratory time – 0.4 sec
Ventilatory rate – 40/min
FiO_2 – 0.75

ABG was done about 20 minutes after ventilation showed:
pH – 7.3
PO_2 – 60 mm Hg (7.8 kPa)
PCO_2 – 35 mm Hg (3.9 kPa)

The baby was pink, but at 10 hours of life the baby suddenly became blue and limp. Management was instituted and within 5 minutes he was back to his active self again.

Give 3 possible causes for the sudden deterioration of the infant.

30. A 4-year-old boy was referred for psychomotor delay and hyperactivity. His mother had normal pregnancy. He was delivered by low forceps. Birth weight 4.3 kg. Apgar score 7 at 1 minute and 10 at 5 minutes. He was well postnatally. Development: he sat at 10 months, walked at 18 months, first word at 2 years, started joining words into sentences at 3 ½years. He had a first cousin (a maternal aunt's son) who had mental retardation of an unknown cause.

Examination:
Cheerful child, broad forehead with elongated ears.
OFC – 53.7cm (father's OFC was 58 cm and mother's was 53 cm)
Fundi: no cherry red spot
CVS, Chest, Abdomen: normal, Testis – 3.5 ml bilaterally.
Neurologically normal Urine: no glucose/albumin.

Investigations:

Serum CPK, T$_4$ normal

Urine – mucopolysaccharides, amino acid, organic acid screen were negative

a)   Mention one investigation to confirm the cause of mental retardation?

b)   What is the most likely diagnosis?

31. A female infant was born to a 23-year old primigravida at 32 weeks of gestation. Birth weight – 1.8 kg. She was asphyxiated at birth but responded well to resuscitation. Apgar 5 at 1 min, 9 at 10 mins, discharged well at 3 weeks of age with weight of 2.1 kg. Child was seen again at 6 weeks of age. Weight was 2.15 kg. Mother was giving her standard infant formula by mixing 9 scoops of formula with 210 ml of water and dividing into 3 feeds a day. She was also supplemented with iron and vitamins.

After making adjustments to the feeds, she was still not thriving, and was put on parenteral nutrition. A week later, her central catheter for parenteral nutrition was removed and pus was noted from the tip. At this moment the child was noted to have swollen left knee. She was afebrile.

a)   Give 3 specific mistakes of the mother's feeding regime?

b)   What is the most likely diagnosis now?

c)   What is the one most important investigation to do to elicit the diagnosis?

32. A 14-year-old girl presented with a 3 weeks history of fever and lethargy on and off. No other significant history. No history of recent travel or contact.

On examination:

Temp – 37.6° C, non toxic, Blood pressure and pulse rate were normal, CVS examination showed a soft systolic murmur.

Investigations:
Hb – 10.2 g/dl
Total count – normal
Blood C and S × 3 negative
Chest X-ray – slight increase in cardiothoracic ratio, otherwise normal
Urine microscopy: no RBC
C and S – normal
She was admitted to the ward, 3 days later, she had sudden development of aphasia.
a) What 2 investigations should be done now?
b) What is the diagnosis?
c) What is the cause of aphasia?

33. A neonate was born at 28 weeks gestation to a diabetic mother, weighing 1.3 kg. The Apgar score was 3 at 1 min and 4 at 5 min after a difficult intubation. She was stabilized on pressures of 20/3, 50 breaths per minute and 45% oxygen, and an umbilical arterial catheter was inserted. She received vitamin K, 0.5 mg intramuscularly, shortly after birth.

Investigations:
Hb – 12 g/dl
Total white cell count – $10 \times 10^9/l$
Platelets – $70 \times 10^9/l$
Na+ – 140 mmol/l
K+ – 4.8 mmol/l
Glucose (BM stix) – <1
pH – 7.05
PCO_2 – 7.8 kPa
PO_2 – 9 kPa
Base deficit – 6
Chest X-ray – bilateral reticular shadowing and air bronchogram.

She had been improving at 83 hours of age when the oxygen saturation dropped suddenly from 90 to 62%, and the mean BP fell from 28 to 15 mm Hg. She required resuscitation with plasma and increased ventilatory support.

Investigations:
Hb – 7.5 g/dl
Total white cell count – 13 × 10^9/l
Platelets – 40 × 109/l
PT – 23 s(control, 12 s)
KPPT – 76 s (control, 25 s)
TT – 20 s (control, 10 s)
pH – 7.21
PCO_2 – 4.9 kPa
PO_2 – 6.6 kPa
Base deficit – 16
Na+ – 122 mmol/l
K+ – 7.3 mmol/l
Urea – 9 mmol/l
Blood glucose – 0.3 mmol/l
Cranial ultrasound scan showed mild ventricular dilatation. Despite all efforts she remained severely hypotensive and hypoglycaemic and died two days later.
a)   What immediate steps were indicated at birth?
b)   What was the cause of her collapse?

34. A 3-month-old boy presented to casualty with recurrent, uncontrolled seizures over the preceding 12 hours. He had 3-4 loose watery stools for the last 3 days for which no specific treatment was given. He was born normally at term, weighing 3.4 kg. He had been recently vaccinated for the first time though pertussis had been excluded. Vaccination had been delayed as a result of maternal anxiety over the death of previous son from pneumonia at the age of 3.5 months. Apart from being treated for recurrent thrush, he had been in good health.

On examination, he was having generalized clonic seizures. His skin turgor was reduced, the pulse was 102 beats per minute and weak. The BP was 105/65 mm of Hg and the heart sounds were normal. The respiratory rate was 75 breaths per minute with moderate intercostal recession and bilateral, scattered inspiratory and expiratory crepitations. The anterior fontanelle was tense and muscle tone generally increased. He had profuse foul smelling semi-solid stools. His condition continued to deteriorate and he passed into coma. He died without gaining consciousness after 3 days.

Investigations:
Hb – 6.5 g/dl
Platelets – 102 × 10⁹/l
Total white cell count – 11 × 10⁹/l
Neutrophils – 10 × 10⁹/l
Na+ – 126 mmol/l
K+ – 2.6 mmol/l
Ca²⁺ – 2.3 mmol/l
Mg²⁺ – 0.6 mmol/l
Glucose – 1.2 mmol/l
Chest X-ray, intertitial infiltrate; over expanded lungs; small heart and narrow mediastinum
Urinalysis, no abnormality detected
CSF, white cells 35 per high power field; protein, 2.3 g/l; glucose – 0.5 mmol/l
a)   What should be included in the child's initial management?
b)   What investigations are included?
c)   What led to the child's death?
d)   What was the underlying diagnosis?

35. A 10-year-old boy was diagnosed to be having small ventricular septal defect at 5 months of age on clinical examination. He was reassured. He lost follow-up because he moved away from the region. He presented this time, after he had fainted during games in school. Had been well prior to this.

On examination:
Looks well
Not in distress. BP – 100/60 mm of Hg, Thrill in the suprasternal notch, heart sounds S1, S2 normal, midsystolic murmur 4/6 over 4th and 5th lower sternal edge, radiating upwards. Early diastolic murmur 1- 2/6 halfway between apex and left sternal edge.
a)   What is the clinical disease?
b)   Name one investigation to guide the severity?

36. A 6-year-old child presented in coma. He was born at term following a normal pregnancy. His initial development revealed that he had good head control at 10 weeks. By then he was able to smile. He sat with support at 8 months and unsupported at 10 months, and walked at 16 months. He babbled and cooed, and he was able to reach out and grasp toys at 8 months. He was able to say six words correctly at 18 months. He had not been taken to child welfare clinic and had not had vitamins at any time. He was artificially fed throughout and solids were introduced at 2 months. He regurgitated his food but this was not serious. He was not seen by a doctor for this symptom.

His parents were poor and they lived with the child in an old house with an outside toilet. He was never immunised and the history revealed that he put everything in his mouth. His bowels were normal and his appetite recently had diminished. Over the previous 6 months, behavioural changes had been noticed.

On admission it was learnt that he had convulsed for approximately 45 minutes before stopping spontaneously.

Examination:
Height – 84 cm (3rd centile)
Weight – 10.7 kg(3rd centile)
Pyrexial – 38°C (axilla)
Pale, not clinically anaemic
Pulse – 112 beats/min; blood pressure– 110/85 mm Hg
Heart sounds normal- no added sounds
Responded to painful stimuli and simple commands
Nuchal rigidity-positive Kernig's sign
Pupils equal, reacted to light
Fundoscopy, early bilateral papilloedema; no haemorrhages or exudates
Diminished tone, upper and lower limbs
Reflexes, sluggish
Plantars, flexor.
a) What is most likely diagnosis?
b) Give two differential diagnoses?
c) Give 3 investigations that you would do as soon as possible?

37. A 14-year-old girl was admitted as an emergency with a three day history of malaise, vomiting and abdominal discomfort. Her general practitioner had found her very drowsy.

On admission she was unarousable, the temperature was 36.8° C and blood pressure was 70/45 mm of Hg.

Investigation:
Plasma sodium – 126 mmol/l
Plasma potassium – 7.0 mmol/l
Plasma chloride – 90 mmol/l
Plasma bicarbonate – 13 mmol/l

Plasma urea – 12 mmol/l
Plasma creatinine – 150 μmol/l
Blood glucose – 1.1 mmol/l
a)   What is the likely diagnosis?
b)   After emergency treatment has been given, what further test would be of most value in confirming the diagnosis?

38. A 5-year-old girl was admitted to hospital with a year's history of recurrent jaundice.
Investigations:
Hb – 11 g/dl
Reticulocytes – 2%
WBC – 10.7 × 10⁹/L
    neutrophils – 5.7 × 10⁹/l
    lymphocytes – 4.3 × 10⁹/l
    monocytes – 0.5 ×10⁹/l
    eosinophils – 0.2 × 10⁹/l
ESR – 10 mm/1st hour (Westergren)
Plasma bilirubin - 65 μmol/l (60 μmol/l conjugated bilirubin)
Serum aspartate aminotransferase (AST) – 70 IU/l (normal range 10-45 IU/l)
Plasma proteins (total) – 60 g/l
Plasma alkaline phosphatase – 500 IU/l (normal range for age 56-190 IU/l)
Urin – Bile + + +
a)   What is the most likely diagnosis?
b)   What further investigation would you do?

39. A girl of 9 years, who had lived all her life in India, presented with marked splenomegaly.
Investigation:
Hb – 6 g/dl
WBC – 2 × 10⁹/L -   neutrophils 0.9 × 10⁹/l
                      lymphocytes 0.6 ×10⁹/l
                      eosinophils 0.1 × 10⁹/l
                      monocytes 0.2 × 10⁹/l

RBC – $2.5 \times 10^{12}/l$
Platelets – $15 \times 10^{9}/l$
ESR – 102 mm/hr
Chest X-ray – normal
Plasma total bilirubin – 6 µmol/l
Plasma albumin – 42 g/l
Plasma globulin – 52 g/l
Plasma alanine aminotransaminase – 38 IU/l (normal range for age 2-12 IU/l)
Plasma aspartate aminotransaminase – 29 IU/l (normal range for age 6-17 IU/l)
Plasma alkaline phosphatase – 270 IU/l (normal range for age 71-177 IU/l)
What is the most likely diagnosis?

40. The following genetic tree is from a family with a genetic disease. Assuming that the gene is not reintroduced into the family by marriage or mutation:

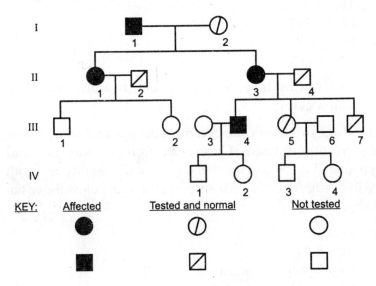

What is the chance that the following individuals will have evidence of the disease?

i)   III 2
ii) IV 1
iii) IV 2
iv) IV 3

41. A girl aged 2 ½ years presented with a history of easy bruising and nose bleeds. She weighed 10 kg, measured 65 cm, with a head circumference of 42 cm, had simple low set ears, vestigial thumbs and scattered areas of increased pigmentation over the trunk.

Investigations:

Hb – 8.9 g/dl
Total white cell count – $3.2 \times 10^9/l$
Platelets – $17 \times 10^9/l$
MCV – 97 fl
MCH – 22 pg
MCHC – 29 g/l
HbA – 79%
HbA_2 – 5%
HbF – 11%

Bone marrow aspirate, reduced cellularity with diminished megakaryocytes

At the age of 4 years she became lethargic and complained of pain in both knees. On examination she was pale and pyrexial. There was generalized lymphadenopathy and both the liver edge and spleen were palpable 3 cm below the costal margin.

Investigations:

Hb – 5.2 g/dl
Total white cell count – $21 \times 10^9/l$
Neutrophils – $1.8 \times 10^9/l$
Platelets – $4 \times 10^9/l$

Bone marrow aspirate, markedly hypercellular marrow
X-ray knees, irregular erosions at the metaphyses
a)   What is the underlying diagnosis?
b)   How could this diagnosis be confirmed?
c)   What remarkable development has occurred at the age
of four?
d)   What is the management for this child?

42. A 3-week-old boy admitted with increasing lethargy and
poor feeding. Born at full term, through spontaneous vertex
delivery, bottlefed, the baby was discharged home on day 5
of life. On day 12 of life he started vomiting, becomes
constipated. On day 19 of life he developed increasing
difficulty in feeding, became more miserable than previously
and at times tended to fight when being fed, vomiting
increased in amounts and the child became more drowsy.
Family history – NAD

Examination:
Jaundice, Temp – 37.5° C, pulse – 135/min, BP – 65/40,
Tachypnoeic – 45-50/min
Hepatosplenomegaly (liver 3 cm, spleen 1 cm)
Anterior fontanelle not buldging

Investigations:
Hb – 14.5 g/dl
TW – 17,500 normal differentials
Platelets – 30,000
Na – 130
K – 4.5
Cl, BU, CSF, Chest X-ray – normal
Urine – no glucose
Culture – no growth
a)   What 2 investigations would you do to assist in
diagnosis?
b)   What is the most probable diagnosis?

43.   A 14-year-old Pakistani girl transferred from a district general hospital for management of status epilepticus after treatment with IV diazepam and IM paraldehyde and IV diazepam infusion. She first started fits at age 4 with fever and subsequently at 4½ years. Both were of short duration. However, on one of her visits to Pakistan, she had convulsed for 5 hours. Following that, her milestones deteriorated. Cause not found despite extensive investigation.

Parents were unsure of her dosage. She has been on primidone, phenytoin and carbamazepine. Occasionally she also requires per rectal diazepam.

Examination now:
She was unresponsive
Still has occasional generalised seizures lasting 2-5 mins
All reflexes depressed
Hypotonia
Fundus: vessels engorged
Pyrexia – 38° C
Crepitations left lower zone and mid zone
BP – 120/80
Investigations:
Hb – 9.0 g/dl
TW – 15,000 normal differentials
Platelets – 300,000
Na – 126
K – 4.5
Normal urea, chloride
Chest X-ray – consolidation left mid zone and left lower zone
On leg X-ray there is fracture of right femur, and the bone looked thin.
a)   Two therapeutic steps you would take now?
b)   Two further investigations to help in management of this girl?

44. A 12-year-old with inflammatory bowel disease and chronic hepatomegaly presented acutely with a temperature of 39.5° C, sweats, rigors and profound lethargy. He had developed mucus diarrhoea 2 days before admission but had become progressively more drowsy with vomiting and right sided abdominal pain. His regular medication included alternate day prednisolone, sulphasalazine and overnight nasogastric feeds. As well as recurrent perianal abscesses, he also suffered with skin boils and chest infections.

On examination he appeared flushed, clammy, poorly perfused, with a heart rate of 120 beats per minute, BP – 105/ 65 mmHg, and a respiratory rate of 32 breaths per minute. Guarding and tenderness were present over the right upper quadrant. The liver edge was palpable 7 cm below the costal margin. The bowel sounds were reduced and there were old healed scars around the anal verge.

Investigations:
Hb – 9.6 g/dl
Total white cell count – 14.8 × 10^9/l
Lymphocytes – 12.3 × 10^9/l
Monocytes – 1.2 × 10^9/l
Platelets – 215 × 10^9/l
ESR – 53 mm in the first hour
Na+ – 132 mmol/l
K+ – 3.2 mmol/l
Urea – 7.4 mmol/l
Creatinine – 0.07 mmol/l
Ca^{2+} – 2.3 mmol/l
Glucose – 1.1mmol/l
AST – 201 U/l
ALT – 157 U/l
Abdominal X-ray, no distended bowel loops, soft tissue shadow in the right upper quadrant.

After 6 hours on intravenous fluids, there was an initial improvement and the lethargy and dizziness improved. This was followed by further deterioration with spiking fevers and worsening abdominal pain.
a) What other investigations are indicated?
b) What has precipitated this admission?
c) What is the underlying condition?

45. A 16-year-old girl is having secondary amenorrhoea. The family spoke very little English and therefore history was difficult to take. She has been taking prednisolone for the last 10 or 15 years in India. She had menses once or twice 2 years ago but not before or subsequent to that. Now she is taking 10 mg of prednisolone. Her weight is 25 kg.

Investigations:
TSH
Prolactin Oestradial – normal
FSH and LH – normal
Progesterone – normal
DHEA – markedly raised
Serum testosterone – raised
17OH progesterone – markedly raised
Urea and electrolytes, LFT, full blood count – normal
a) What endocrine abnormality is present?
b) What else would you prescribe?
c) What are the two possible explanations for her amenorrhoea?

46. A 12-year-old girl presented with sudden onset of blindness of her right eye. She had injury of her big toe two weeks ago.

Examination:
Low grade temperature
Right eye: blind, loss of red light reflex, disc pale, tortuous, vessels, blotchy? Haemorrhage

Paronychia of the right toe, painful on pressing pulp
Ejection systolic murmur 2/6 at the base of heart
Lungs and abdomen – normal

Investigations:
Urine microscopy and culture: some red cells, no protein or white blood cells
Full blood count – normal
Us and Es – normal
Liver function tests – normal
ESR – normal
Chest X-ray – normal
a)   Name 2 helpful diagnostic investigations?
b)   What is the diagnosis?
c)   What is the cause of the blindness in the right eye?

47. A 14-year-old West Indian girl with 6 months history of lethargy and dark coloured urine with normal coloured stool. She had rubella vaccination one week prior to the onset. Initially she had flu like symptoms after the immunisation. Three weeks later she developed jaundice, fever, and abdominal pain for two days. Jaundice persisted. Vomited for many times a day for one week. Subsequently the vomiting subsided but the anorexia continued for another 3-4 months.
Father had polyarthritis, treated with steroid.

Examination:
Jaundiced. Normal height and weight
Liver and spleen not palpable
No evidence of chronic liver disease
No rashes or hirsutism

Investigations:
Serum bilirubin – raised, mainly unconjugated
Aspartate transaminase, alanine transaminase, alkaline phosphatase – moderately raised

Albumin – low 25
Immunoglobulin was markedly raised
Prothrombin time, partial thromboplastin time – slightly more than control
Urine bile pigment present
Hepatitis A and B serology – ve
Ultrasound – gall bladder contracted. Bile duct not dilated but the patient didn't fast prior to ultrasound. Liver looking normal. Cyst posterior to right kidney.
a)   Name 2 other investigations that may help you in your diagnosis?
b)   What causes jaundice?

48. A known asthmatic, well controlled on oral theophylline, presented with cough and fever and wheezing. He was admitted because he became more dyspnoeic and wheezing persisted.
Hb – 9.9 g/dl
TWDC – 4.5 × 10^9
40% N, 45% L
Platelets – 100,000
What is the diagnosis other than asthma?

49. A 10-year-old boy with cystic fibrosis on ciprofloxacin prophylaxis. Admitted one month for two weeks course of IV flucloxacillin because of staphylococcal infection of the lung. At this time because of right knee pain, fever and cough for 3 days.

Examination:
Febrile
Eczema behind both knees
Right knee red, painful swollen with limited movement
Lungs: basal crackles

Chest X-ray – patchy opacity both lung field with consolidation at left lower lobe
a)   Give 2 investigations you would do immediately to help in your diagnosis.
b)   What is your diagnosis?

50. A 2-week-old baby admitted with 48 hours of vomiting after every feed. On admission she is dehydrated and there is no abdominal distension. Nasogastric aspirate showed 90 mls of greenish aspirate. Abdominal X-ray done on admission showed a distended stomach and fluid level with no gas beyond duodenum. She was treated with IV dextrose – saline and nasogastric aspiration.
After 24 hours another X-ray was repeated with 50 cc of air injected into the stomach. The fluid level has disappeared and gas shadow has gone lower down.
a)   What is the diagnosis?
b)   What one investigation would you do other than correcting the dehydration?

1. a) Guillain-Barre syndrome
   b) Serial peak flow
   Clue: Symmetrical flaccid paraplegia.
   Discussion: In a gray case it is most important to pick up the most important problem. The most important problem in this case is flaccid paraplegia. Any flaccid paraplasia in the developed world without sensory involvement is Guillain-Barre unless proved otherwise. The paralysis in the case discussed is symmetrical which strengthens the diagnosis.

   Involvement of arms makes us cautious of the most dangerous situation of GB syndrome—the diaphragmatic involvement. Therefore, serial peak flow will get priority as the next important investigation to nerve conduction velocity. Nerve conduction velocity may a diagnostic aid but not of great practical value in management. The philosophy of this exam is towards practical approach to solve the patients problems not the theoretical excellence.

2. a) Crohn's disease.
   b) Colonoscopy and biopsy.
   Clues – Weight loss, abdominal pain.
   Discussion: It is important to pick up clues in the history. When we get a constellation of abdominal pain, erythema nodosum, aphthous ulcers, and raised ESR with weight loss, we should think of inflammatory bowel disease. One should remember that growth or pubertal failure by itself is a very important manifestation of these conditions especially at around the age of 15. Other important causes of growth failure at this age may be coeliac disease and Turner's syndrome. But these won't present with aphthous ulcer or erythema nodosum. It is important to know that some of the eating disorders like

anorexia nervosa can mimic Crohn's disease and can be associated with it.

3. a) Nephrotic syndrome
    b) Hypovolemia
    Clues – Oedema, albuminuria.
    Discussion: Main issue here is the oedema. Whenever there is oedema, one should look at the albumin. Whenever, there is low albumin we should try to find out from where this albumin is lost. If it is lost from the intestine, we should consider the diagnosis of protein-losing enteropathy due to intestinal lymphangiectasia. If it is lost in the urine, we should think of nephrotic syndrome.

    If the values of Na, K, Urea is given one should calculate osmolality 2(Na+K)+Urea+ Glucose.

    Here we can assume that the value of glucose to be normal. If osmolality is high as in this case, in a child with nephrotic syndrome, the likely cause of deterioration of renal function is hypovolemia.

4. a) RDS
    b) Congestive cardiac failure.
    Discussion: Respiratory distress that develops within 4 hours of age in a preterm baby is RDS.
    Cause of respiratory problem in a baby who had cord prolapse and perinatal asphyxia is congestive cardiac failure unless proved otherwise.

5. a) Blood culture
    b) Meningococcal sepsis
    c) 1. Fluid therapy
        2. Antibiotics

Discussion: Whenever there is vasculitic rash of acute onset, one should think of the diagnosis of meningococcal sepsis. This type of rash can also occur in collagen vascular disease. However, as meningococcal disease is a life threatening condition, it is important to think of it first, prior to any other diagnosis.

6. a) Guillain-Barre syndrome
    b) Intubation and ventilation
    Discussion: In a gray case it is most important to pick up the most important problem. The most important problem in this case is flaccid paraplegia. Any flaccid paraplasia in the developed world without sensory involvement is Guillain-Barre unless proved otherwise. The paralysis in the case discussed is symmetrical which strengthens the diagnosis.

    Involvement of arms makes us cautious of the most dangerous situation of GB syndrome—the diaphragmatic involvement. Therefore, serial peak flow will get priority as the next important investigation to nerve conduction velocity. Nerve conduction velocity may a diagnostic aid but not of great practical value in management. The philosophy of this exam is towards practical approach to solve the patients problems not the theoretical excellence.

7. Group B streptococcal sepsis.
    Discussion: Respiratory distress syndrome like picture in a term baby without maternal diabetes makes us think of GBS sepsis. Inborn error of metabolism and transient tachypnoea can cause similar picture but X-ray will not show typical ground glass appearance.

8. a) Visual field testing
    b) Lateral X-ray of the skull, CT scan, bone age.
    c) Craniopharyngioma
    Discussion: Growth and pubertal failure can occur due to a variety of causes. As this boy's growth was normal till the age of 8 years, growth hormone deficiency—a common cause of short stature becomes unlikely. This child's general health has been good and appetite has been normal. This rules out common systemic causes like coeliac disease and inflammatory bowel disease. However, this child has a long standing morning headache. This points out towards an intracranial pathology. Craniopharyngioma is a common benign tumour of the brain, causing growth and pubertal failure. Children with craniopharyngioma may have visual field defect, which can give a clinical clue towards the diagnosis. Skull X-ray and CT scan can show evidence of calcification.

9. a) Bronchiectasis due to primary ciliary dyskinesia.
    b) CT chest
    c) Ciliary Mortility Study Nasal potential difference.
    Discussion: Clue lies in recurrent chest infection and failure to thrive to make us think of differential diagnosis cystic fibrosis also. However, sweat test is normal. Furthermore, a CF child will have more pronounced failure to thrive.

10. a) Bronchoalveolar lavage for *Pneumocystis carinii.*
    b) HIV serology
    c) IV cotrimoxazole
        IV amphotericin B.
    Clue– African origin.

Discussion: Oral candidiasis-in a 4-month old suggests immunodeficiency. This is further supported by cervical lymphadenopathy and hepatosplenomegaly, SCID (Subacute combine immunodeficiency) may be an acceptable answer for early presentation of immunodeficiency. However, mother being African, we must think of HIV first – HIV being so common in Africa.

11. a) Munchausen syndrome by proxy.
     b) Urine and serum osmolality profiles off DDAVP with mother absent.

Discussion: Concentrated urine even when DDAVP was not given, rules out diabetes insipidus. Mother was diluting and manipulating the previous urine samples.

12. a) FBC, Coagulation Screen
     b) Blood transfusion, fresh frozen plasma
     c) Haemorrhagic disease of newborn due to vitamin K deficiency.

Clue- Exclusively breastfed baby.

Discussion: Sticky stool in a 4-day old breast fed baby makes us suspect of haemorrhagic disease of newborn. As the child is pale and in shock, blood transfusion may be effective. Fresh frozen plasma and not Vitamin K is effective in stopping blood loss acutely.

13. a) Sweat test
     b) Cystic fibrosis
     c) Meconium ileus equivalent

Clues–Clubbing, respiratory illness, malabsorption.

Discussion: Clubbing in a Caucasian boy strongly-suggests cystic fibrosis (CF) unless proved otherwise. Diarrhoea with respiratory illness strengthens this diagnosis to other causes of diarrhoea and malabsorption. Coeliac is an important cause of mal-absorption causing bulky stool. However, jejunal biopsy is normal and respiratory signs are present to rule out coeliac.

14. a) Ultrasonogram hip, bone scan, blood culture
    b) Retrocaecal appendicitis
    Clue–Hip internally rotated and flexed and not externally rotated and extended.
    Discussion: Abdominal pain can radiate to the hip, mimicking hip pathology and vice versa just like chest pain can radiate to abdomen and vice versa. In primary hip pathology hip will be in a position of extension and external rotation, the position of maximum space.

15. a) Dermatomyositis
    b) Muscle biopsy
    Discussion: Muscle weakness with rash is derma-tomyositis. Only muscle weakness would have been polymyositis.

16. a) G6PD, Hepatitis
    b) Haemoglobinuria, bilirubinuria
    Clue s–Turkish, Cypriot origin.

17. a) Tumor lysis syndrome, prerenal failure
    b) Blood film, bone marrow
    c) Acute lymphoblastic leukaemia
    Clue – Pancytopaenia, raised uric acid.
    Discussion: Whenever we have an investigation, in our case history, we should look at it first. This is pancytopenic picture. This may occur in acute leukaemia and aplastic anaemia. As acute lymphoblastic leukaemia is more common, that should be the likely cause. Here,

it is important to understand that the commonest differential diagnosis is always the best answer.

18. a) Rupture of bronchial collateral due to pulmonary hypertension.
    b) Atrial fibrillation
    c) Infective endocarditis
    d) Pulmonary embolism
    Discussion: Loud P2 and cyanosis in a child with VSD indicates pulmonary hypertension. There is ankle oedema, raised JVP, and crackles in the chest signifying heart failures. Heart failures is unusual with pulmonary hypertension. However, if there is infective endocarditis there may be heart failure, even if there is pulmonary hypertension. Atrial fibrillation can be an additional cause of heart failure causing deterioration of the symptoms.

19. a) Hereditary spherocytosis or congenital haemolytic anaemia.
    b) Autohaemolysis tests.
    c) Hypoplastic crisis secondary to parvovirus infection.
    Discussion: Autohaemolysis compared to osmotic fragility, is becoming a more popular diagnostic test in hereditary spherocytosis.

20. Congenital cyanotic heart disease- transposition of great arteries (TGA).
    Persistent foetal hypertension.
    Clues – Metabolic acidosis, cyanosis in early newborn period.
    Discussion: Metabolic acidosis with cyanosis in newborn baby should make us think of congenital cyanotic heart disease, TGA (being commonest) and persistent foetal

hypertension. RDS will produce respiratory acidosis. This is a common exam scenario.

21. a) Urinary catecholamines, MIBG scan, bone marrow
    b) Neuroblastoma
    Clue –Right hypochondrium (suprarenal mass).
    Discussion: Suprarenal mass and liver metastasis is common in neuroblastoma.

22. Reactive arthritis.
    Clue –Viral illness, Joint pain.
    Discussion: Reactive arthritis is very common. The preceding viral type of illness, normal ESR, bone scan and hip X-ray points out towards that.

23. a) Toxic shock syndrome
    b) 1) Streptococci, 2) Staphylococci, 3) Infected vaginal tampoons
    Clues–Sudden onset of fever and hypotension in postpubertal girl.
    Discussion: Sudden onset of fever, rash and hypotension is suggestive of toxic shock syndrome. Toxic-shock syndrome, haemorrhagic shock syndrome and Kawasaki disease are common topics in exam. Differential diagnosis of toxic shock syndrome is meningococcal disease.

24. a) Blood culture, joint fluid aspiration and culture
    b) Pneumococcal septic arthritis
    c) Pneumococcal vaccine
        Penicillin prophylaxis.
    Clue – Arthritis in a spleenotomised boy.

Discussion: Post splenectomy pneumococcal infection are common in haemolytic anaemia. Other issues that are examiner's favourites are gall stones causing right upper abdominal pain and pneumonia and sickle chest syndrome in sickle cell anaemia.

25. a) Laryngospasm
    b) Anaphylaxis
    c) O_2
       IM adrenaline

Discussion: IM adrenaline and not IV is treatment of choice according to latest Advanced Paediatric Life Support guidelines for anaphylaxis.

26. a) Echocardiogram
    b) Kawasaki disease.
    Clues–Fever, cervical lymphoedema, rash, conjunctivitis, erythema of hands, high platelet count.

Discussion: Red herring like appearance of rash after starting amoxycillin is very common exam scenario and should not deviate one from main issues.

27. a) Ultrasound abdomen
       Right hip joint fluid aspiration cytology and culture
    b) Septic arthritis right hip
       Psoas abscess.

Discussion: The flexed position of the hip makes us suspect the abdominal pathology. Though hip pathology cannot be ruled out, the flexed position of hip is not the position that provides maximum space.

Blood culture and bone scan can also be a probable answer to the question.

28. a) Idiopathic precocious puberty

b) CT scan
Bone age: Left wrist X-ray
FSH, LH cortisol
Clue –Precocious puberty in a girl is idiopathic unless proved otherwise.
Discussion: Tall stature, with early breast and pubic hair development is a feature of precocious puberty. As there is consonance (development of all secondary sexual characters in order), it is true precocious puberty. A true precocious puberty in a girl is idiopathic unless proved otherwise.

29. Displaced tube
Obstructed tube
Pneumothorax
Equipment failure
Discussion: Whenever there is a sudden deterioration of a newborn baby being ventilated think about DOPE.
D – displaced tube
O – obstructed tube
P – pneumothorax
E – equipment failure
This is a common exam scenario, as in practical life.

30. a) DNA studies for trinucleotide repeat.
b) Fragile X syndrome
Discussion: Fragile X syndrome is the second common cause of learning disability, after Down's syndrome. Prevalence is 1 in 1000 to 2500. Macro-orchidism and big ear are the dysmorphic features; others are generally soft.

31. a) More concentrated feeds. 9 scoops in 270 mls
Less feeds
Less number of feeds

    b) Septic arthritis

    c) Bone scan

Discussion: Commonest cause of failure to thrive is faulty feeding. Long lines are notorious for infections.

32. a) Echocardiogram, CT scan of head

    b) Subacute bacterial endocarditis

    c) Embolism

Discussion: Neurologic manifestation in a child with systolic murmur is likely to be secondary to embolism following infective endocarditis.

33. a) Blood culture

      Urine for reducing substances

    b) Inborn error of metabolism, probably galactosaemia

Discussion: Poor feeding, lethargy, vomiting and jaundice in a newborn with or without convulsion may be a feature of either sepsis or inborn error of metabolism. Fluctuation of manifestation with inborn error of metabolism is very much related to stopping and starting of feeds. Hepatosplenomegaly and jaundice in a baby with inborn error of metabolism is commonly due to galactosaemia. Note that though glucose in urine is negative, reducing substance in the urine would have been positive. Galactosaemia can sometimes present like Fanconi's syndrome. *E. coli* sepsis is common in galactosemic patients.

34. a) Treatment of raised intracranial pressure and seizures, pneumonia, anaemia, hypoglycaemia, hyponatraemia and hypokalaemia.

    b) T-cells subsets, immunoglobulins, stool and CSF virology, blood culture, blood gas.

c) Polio virus encephalitis

d) Severe combined immunodeficiency

Discussion: Live polio vaccination can cause disseminated disease in immunodeficiency states, SCID can present earlier than other causes of common immunodeficiency syndrome. Encephalitis can cause SIADH leading to low sodium.

35. a) Aortic stenosis with aortic regurgitation

b) Echocardiogram

Clues- Fainting, suprasternal thrill, diastolic murmur.

Discussion: The fainting and the suprasternal thrill points towards AS. Diastolic murmur points towards regurgitation.

36. a) Lead encephalopathy

b) Viral encephalitis, space occupying lesion.

c) Blood lead level

Urinary coproporphyrins

CT or MRI scan

Discussion: Lead encephalopathy should always be considered in cases of unexplained encephalopathy. Furthermore, the child in our case is not so well preserved child with history of pica beyond the age of physiologic pica. Papilloedema may be a sign of lead encephalopathy.

37. a) Acute adrenal insufficiency

b) Synacthen test

Clues–Hyponatraemia, hyperkalaemia, low glucose

Discussion: Hyponatraemia and hyperkalaemia points towards adrenal failure, either an acute failure or in form of Addison's disease and congenital adrenal hyperplasia.

38. a) Choledochal cyst.
    b) Abdominal ultrasonogram.
    Clues–Recurrent jaundice, conjugated hyperbiliru-
    binaemia
    Discussion: Recurrent jaundice with high conjugated
    bilirubin and bile in urine, points towards choledochal
    cyst. If this was recurrent mild jaundice with mainly
    unconjugated bilirubin, it is Gilbert's Disease—a mild
    condition.

39. Kala azar
    Clues–Pancytopenia, splenomegaly, India
    Discussion: Isolated splenomegaly in a Caucasian child
    is hereditary spherocytosis unless proved otherwise.
    Similarly, isolated splenomegaly in an Indian population
    can be chronic haemolytic anaemia, myloid leukaemia
    and kala azar. However, pancytopenic picture points
    more towards kala azar.

40. i) 50%
    ii) 0%
    iii) 100%
    iv) 0%
    Clues–All generations affected
    No male to male transmission.
    Discussion: As all generations are affected, the scenario
    points towards dominant inheritance.
    As there is no male to male transmission apparent, this
    is more likely to be X-linked.
    In X-linked dominant inheritance all daughters of the
    affected male is affected as the X chromosome from male
    is transmitted to their daughters but not to their sons.
    The affected X chromosome from the mother are
    transmitted both to the female and male equally and
    there is 50% chance of transmission to either sex.

41. a) Fanconi's anaemia
    b) White cell chromosome fragility test
    c) Acute myeloid leukaemia
    d) Supportive antibiotics, blood and platelet trans-
        fusions, chemotherapy.

    Discussion: Constellation of pancytopenia , high MCV
    and HbF, short stature with dysmorphic feature, makes
    the diagnosis of Fanconi's anaemia as like other
    conditions with chromosomal fragility, childrens' with
    Fanconi's anaemia are more prone for malignancies,
    commonest of which is AML.

42. a) Gal-put test
        Clinitest
    b) Galactosaemia

    Clues–Bottlefed baby getting worse.
    Investigation suggestive of sepsis.
    Jaundice
    Hepatosplenomegaly.

    Discussion: Features of sepsis like poor feeding,
    vomiting, lethargy and convulsion should make us alert
    about inborn error of metabolism, which often improves
    after withdrawal of feeds.

    Investigations suggestive of sepsis in an otherwise
    likely case of inborn error of metabolism should make
    us alert of galactosaemia where *E. coli* sepsis is common.
    Jaundice and hepatosplenomegaly are also suggestive
    of galactosaemia. It is important that galactosaemia can
    present like Fanconi's syndrome and a Fanconi like
    picture in the exam situation should make us think of
    galactosaemia.

    A close differential diagnosis is organic acidaemia
    and, therefore, urinary organic acid estimation may also
    be an acceptable answer.

43. a) IPPV Mannitol
        IV calcium
    b) Drug levels
        Ca, Phosphorus, alkaline phosphatase
    Clues–Phenytoin use, pathological fracture
    Discussion: Pathological fracture in a child with
    unresponsive status epilepticus makes us think of
    hypocalcaemia. CT scan head also could have been a
    relevant answer to question b.

44. a) Blood cultures, abdominal ultrasound scan.
    b) Liver or subdiaphragmatic abscess
    c) Type Ib glycogen storage disease.
    Discussion: Inflammatory bowel disease may be
    associated with some glycogen storage disease and other
    inborn errors of metabolism. The glucose level is likely
    to be low and liver is enlarged if there is coexisting
    glycogen storage disease with inflammatory bowel
    disease. Because of immunosuppressive therapy of
    inflammatory bowel disease, abscess in the enlarged liver
    can occur.

45. a) Congenital adrenal hyperplasia
    b) Fludrocortisone acetate.
    c) Relative decrease of oestrogen due to increase in
        testosterone
    Inadequate steroid treatment, excessive androgen, poor
    compliance.
    Discussion: Raised hydroxyprogesterone activity is due
    to congenital adrenal hyperplasia which can present with
    amenorrhoea and excessive virilisation in girls.

46. a) Blood culture
        Echocardiogram

b) Bacterial endocarditis
c) Embolic manifestation
Clues–Sudden onset of blindness
Systolic murmur
Discussion: Commonest cause of sudden onset of blindness in childhood is embolic manifestation. The commonest cause of embolic manifestation in a child is SBE.

47. a) Autoantibody screen
    Liver biopsy
    b) Chronic active hepatitis
    Clues–High immunoglobulin
    West Indian girl
    Discussion: Autoimmune process with single or multiple system affection is common among girls compared to boys and more common in Afro-Caribbean ancestry. Sickle cell disease with gall stone is a close differential. However, raised immunoglobulin and absence of gall stones make it less likely.

48. Mycoplasma pneumonia
    Clues–Anaemia
    Thrombocytopenia
    Discussion: Asthma like respiratory illness with anaemia and thrombocytopenia makes us suspicious of Mycoplasma infection. Even some cases of poorly controlled asthma become well controlled after a course of erythromycin.

49. a) Blood culture
    Knee joint aspiration cytology and culture
    b) Septic arthritis
    Pneumonia

Clue–Arthritis involving one joint.

Discussion: Though Ciprofloxacin causes arthropathy, by far the most important cause of arthritis is involving one joint is septic arthritis. It is important to note however that nonspecific arthritis can occur in CF, due to high levels of circulating immune complex. Vasculitis causing joint pain can also occur in association with advanced lung disease.

50. a) Intermittent volvulous due to malrotation.
    b) Barium meal.

Discussion: Intermittent intestinal obstruction in the newborn period is a feature of malrotation.

Index

A

Abdominal pain 24, 62, 80, 81
Abnormal movements 26
Abscess 13
Absence seizure 45
Achondroplasia 19
Acute leukaemia 31
Acute lymphoblastic leukaemia 89
Acute renal failure 40
Adenosine 42
Adrenal failure 95
Amenorrhoea 11
Anaemia 14, 37
Anaphylaxis 92
Aneuria 29
Aortic stenosis 95
Aphasia 69
Aplastic anaemia 39
Arthritis 91
Aspirin 41
Asthma 82
Atrial fibrillation 90
Audiogram 22

B

Backache 51
Bacterial meningitis 31
Barium meal 100
Blood gas 6, 8, 24
Blood sugar 44
Bloody diarrhoea 18, 38
Bronchiectasis 87
Bronchoalveolar lavage 87
Bruising 61, 76
Bruit 3

C

Cardiomegaly 63, 91
Cardiovascular disease 11
Cerebral abscess 31
Cervical lymphadenopathy 57
Chest pain 61
Choledochal cyst 96
Clubbing 5
Coeliac disease 36
Compensated respiratory acidosis 44
Congenital adrenal hyperplasia 98
Congenital cyanotic heart disease 90
Congestive cardiac failure 85
Conjugated bilirubin 74
Convulsion 5, 9
Cough 7, 10, 14, 56, 58, 62, 82
Crohn's disease 84
Cyanosis 62, 67, 90
Cystic fibrosis 38, 82
Cystinosis 46
Cystinuria 47

D

Deafness 10
Dehydration 12
Diabetes insipidus 57
Diabetes mellitus 37
Diamond-Blackfan syndrome 41
Diarrhoea 21, 25, 26, 63
Diastolic murmur 72
Dilatation of renal pelvis 27
Down's syndrome 12, 36, 42

Duchenne-muscular dystrophy 43
Dyspnoea 14

E

ECG 4, 6, 11, 19, 26
Eczema 56
Embolism 94
Epilepsy 56
Erythema nodosum 51, 84
Excessive thirst 57

F

Facial swelling 52
Fanconi's anaemia 97
Fanconi's syndrome 46, 94
Fever 10, 18, 51, 53, 63, 64, 68, 81, 82
Flaccid paraplegia 84
Fludrocortisone acetate 98
Foetal hypertension 90
Folic acid deficiency 36
Fragile X syndrome 93

G

Galactosaemia 97
Genetic disease 75
Gluten free diet 43
Goitre 4
Guillain-Barre syndrome 84, 86

H

Haematuria 15
Haemolytic uraemic syndrome
     37
Haemoptysis 61
Headache 53
Heart failure 5
Heart murmur 17
Hepatitis 99
Hepatomegaly 79
Hepatosplenomegaly 77
Hereditary spherocytosis 34, 90

Hyperkalaemia 46
Hyperuricaemia 31
Hypocalcaemia 31
Hypokalaemia 46
Hypoparathyroidism 32
Hypothyroidism 30
Hypovolemia 85
Hypoxia 33

I

Inflammatory bowel disease 79
Iron deficiency 33
Iron deficiency anaemia 38

J

Jaundice 12, 25, 26, 74, 81

K

Kala-azar 96
Karyotype 15, 17
Kawasaki disease 92
Ketotic hypoglycaemia 34

L

Lead encephalopathy 95
Lethargy 61, 68, 77, 79, 81
Lumps in the groin 5

M

Malaise 51, 73
Meningitis 65
Mental retardation 67
Munchausen syndrome 88
Mycoplasma pneumonia 99
Myocardial infarction 9

N

Neck stiffness 10
Nephrotic syndrome 33
Night sweats 51

O

Ostium primum 30
Otitis media 56

P

Panhypopituitarism 44
Paracetamol overdose 44
Penicillin prophylaxis 91
Pertussis 58, 70
Pharyngeal ulcers 51
Photophobia 5
Pneumococcal vaccine 91
Polydipsia 34
Polyuria 34, 57
Precocious puberty 92
Proteinuria 52
Pubertal growth spurt 45
Pulmonary atresia 32
Pulmonary embolism 90
Pulmonary stenosis 30
Purpura 15
Pyrexia 5, 76

R

Rash 53, 60, 63, 64
Renal colic 29
Renal failure 61
Renal glycosuria 38
Respiratory distress 8, 55, 67
Respiratory distress syndrome 32, 33
Respiratory tract infections 51
Retrocaecal appendicitis 89
Rickets 38, 41, 45
Right iliac fossa mass 59
Rigors 79

S

Scrotal oedema 52

Seizures 70
Sensorineural deafness 43
Septic arthritis 94, 99
Short stature 11, 23
Small stature 55
Smoky urine 8
Splenomegaly 74
Stridor 7, 64
Subdiaphragmatic abscess 98
Sudden onset of blindness 80
Supraventricular tachycardia 42
Sweat test 44, 88
Synacthen test 95
Systemic lupus erythematosus 42
Systolic bruit 3
Systolic murmur 6

T

Tetralogy of Fallot 43
Tonsillectomy 14
Toxic shock syndrome 91
Tuberculous meningitis 30, 35
Turner's syndrome 40, 84

V

Viral encephalitis 95
Vomiting 5, 10, 17, 24, 26, 57, 63, 64, 73, 77
von Willebrand's disease 40

W

Waddling gait 18
Wheeze ·7, 82
Whooping cough 39
Wolff-Parkinson-White (WPW) syndrome 32

X

X-linked recessive 43